ALCHEMICAL
TANTRIC
ASTROLOGY

★ ★ ★

"*Alchemical Tantric Astrology* is a profound marriage of three sets of symbols. They all come together as the serpent fully uncoils at the crown, unveiled by the Moon's nodes. Hermes's signposts on the way to self-realization light them up as never before! Creative and original—not to be missed!"

MICHAEL BURTON, PH.D.,
LICENSED ACUPUNCTURIST AND
LICENSED ASTROLOGICAL COUNSELOR

"A unique and useful integration of cosmology, chakras and metals, spiritual yoga, and meditations."

PRATIBHA GRAMANN, PH.D., TRANSCENDENTAL
PSYCHOLOGIST, SCHOLAR, YOGA THERAPIST,
AND AYURVEDA EDUCATOR

"Frederick Baker's wit and scholarly approach emboss a brilliant and highly original formation that holds great promise for all students of astrology and yoga."

NANCY KURTZ, ASTROLOGER

"Speaking in symbols we discuss a shared truth that is deeper than words can describe. When we can see solid, clear intersections across symbolic systems, we see truths deeper than any system alone could say. Frederick Baker has given us this, through his blessed lifelong focus, a new weave of our oldest views of the 'beyond verbal,' weaving those shared beauties into a yet deeper view of our reality."

MICHAEL BARTLOW, PIANIST,
COMPOSER, AND WRITER

ALCHEMICAL TANTRIC ASTROLOGY

The Hidden Order of Seven Metals, Seven Planets, and Seven Chakras

A Sacred Planet Book

FREDERICK HAMILTON BAKER

Destiny Books
Rochester, Vermont

Destiny Books
One Park Street
Rochester, Vermont 05767
www.DestinyBooks.com

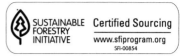

Text stock is SFI certified

Destiny Books is a division of Inner Traditions International

Sacred Planet Books are curated by Richard Grossinger, Inner Traditions editorial board member and cofounder and former publisher of North Atlantic Books. The Sacred Planet collection, published under the umbrella of the Inner Traditions family of imprints, is comprised of works on the themes of consciousness, cosmology, alternative medicine, dreams, climate, permaculture, alchemy, shamanic studies, oracles, astrology, crystals, hyperobjects, locutions, and subtle bodies.

Cataloging-in-Publication Data for this title is available from the Library of Congress

ISBN 978-1-64411-280-9 (print)
ISBN 978-1-64411-281-6 (ebook)

Printed and bound in the United States by Lake Book Manufacturing, Inc. The text stock is SFI certified. The Sustainable Forestry Initiative® program promotes sustainable forest management.

10   9   8   7   6   5   4   3   2   1

Text design and layout by Virginia Scott Bowman
This book was typeset in Garamond Premier Pro and Gill Sans with Acherous Grotesque and Carentro used as display typefaces

Alchemical Tantric Arrangement, chakra, and zodiac artwork by Bruce Harman
Astrology charts were created using TimePassages by AstroGraph Software, Inc. (www.astrograph.com)

To send correspondence to the author of this book, mail a first-class letter to the author c/o Inner Traditions • Bear & Company, One Park Street, Rochester, VT 05767, and we will forward the communication, or contact the author directly at **www.alchemicaltantricastrology.com.**

♦♦♦

I dedicate this book to you,
Jane Ellen Harrison,
scholar, feminist, and psychologically savvy
British mythologist: it's more than a century later
and you are still way ahead of the pack! All I can say is:
wow, and thanks!

Benediction

Praise to you, dear Galaxy of the brilliant Milky Way, reaching out sparkling spiraling arms from your massive pulsating heart center. You are the dark central Great Goddess of Night and Light, spraying starry milk from your breasts. Gazing heavenward, your divine femininity is always included in my night vision.

Likewise, I honor you, Great Goddess, as Greek mother and midwife Maia, of the dark cave and night sky, who gave birth to your trickster son Hermes, later called Mercurius. Magnificent Maia, your name is given to one of the star gals of the Pleiades, the Seven Sisters.

Mother Maia, you are in my mind connected to the Mesoamerican star-watching Maya, the Hindu goddess Maya of the swirling phenomenal world, and Maya mother of the Buddha, who is also the planet Mercury and thus your son Hermes . . . all thanks be to you.

Contents

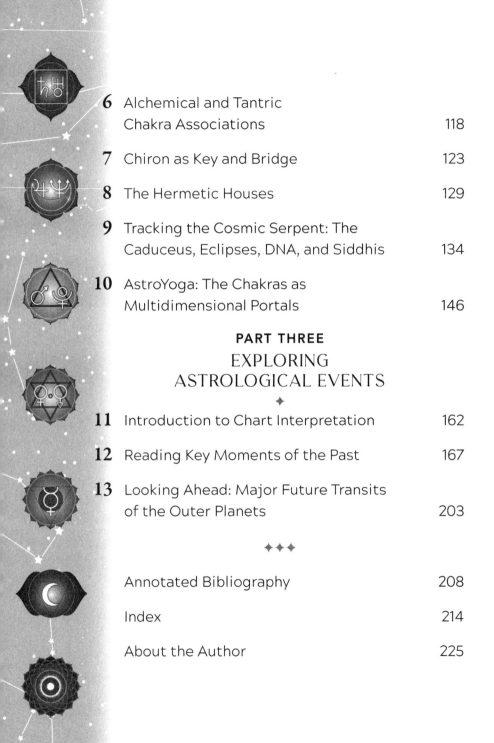

PART THREE
EXPLORING
ASTROLOGICAL EVENTS
✦

✦ ✦ ✦

Acknowledgments

I have been blessed with amazing teachers throughout my life. In the context of this book, I give special thanks to three teachers I have had the great good fortune to meet in person: Dane Rudhyar, humanistic astrologer; James Hillman, archetypal psychologist; and Baba Hari Dass, Himalayan yogi. They have profoundly affected the contents of this book. I also thank the Cosmic Choreographer who gracefully brought information and experiences at just the right time.

The following folks are also directly related to the contents of this book, and so a huge thanks goes out to them: Jeannine Parvati, Suzuki Roshi, Terence McKenna, John Major Jenkins, Prasanna, Tara, Norman O. Brown, Ganapati Sthapati, Ronald Quinn, Ronald L. Byrnes, and Bruce Harman.

It took a long time to get to the point of having the completed book that you are now reading; however, it came together rather painlessly with great support from Richard Grossinger and all the very talented and highly professional publishers at Inner Traditions • Bear & Company. My lovely and brilliant wife, Judith Claire Joy, has read the book over and over and over for many years while helping edit the manuscript and has somehow stayed positive and super helpful.

I want to thank the two grandfathers after whom I was named: Frederick, a 33rd degree Mason who took me on a dream tour through the Great Pyramid, and Hamilton, a Wyoming country doctor. And my parents, Helen and Hugh, and all the teachers, friends, and family who have put up with my egocentric antics all these years.

The Holy Cross and the Labyrinth

This brief historical account is meant to clarify how the ideas contained in this book have developed.

I moved to Santa Cruz (Holy Cross), California, in 1965 as Uranus became conjunct with Pluto and as they were transiting the first house of my natal chart. Considering, as you'll discover, that the alchemical elements associated with these two planets are uranium and plutonium, an astrologer might conclude that some explosive changes might be in store on an identity level, the first house being related to basic identity.

And indeed, major shifts were in store. Dropping my dentistry program, I chose to attend the new campus of the University of California, Santa Cruz, instead. Shortly thereafter, I met Suzuki Roshi at UCSC and began Zen meditation. Soon after that, I got my first astrology reading from Santa Cruz iconic astrologer Lew Fein and began studying the subject with a passion. I was drawn to the psychological writings of C. G. Jung, including his work on astrology and alchemy. It was around this same time that I read the classic account of alchemy by Titus Burckhardt, *Alchemy: Science of the Cosmos, Science of the Soul*. This book laid the basic foundation for the connections between alchemy and astrology, as the following quote makes clear:

Alongside the planetary hierarchy which is inversely related to that of the metals, there is also another and older ordering of the planets which runs parallel to the alchemical order. This is their gradation according to "houses," the distribution of which in the zodiac only becomes meaningful when their common axis is situated in the way in which, in all probability, it was situated in the original zodiac of about two thousand years before Christ. At that time the axis of the solstice passed between Leo and Cancer at the upper end, so that, as a result, the so-called planetary houses became symmetrically arranged. As Julius Schwabe has shown, *there is much to suggest that this position of the heavens was fundamental for all astrological symbolism.* [Emphasis mine]

Burckhardt goes on to almost, but not quite, make the connection of the seven metals and seven planets arranged in the seven houses to the seven chakras when he shows an image of the "seven shakras" in the context of what he calls the "primordial serpent" in the "Tantric representation."*

There is no doubt that this book on alchemy made a lasting impression on me, waiting many years in the back of my psyche for a return to this present connection of alchemy and astrology to the tantric yoga chakra system.

From 1968 to 1970, the U.S. Navy helped me take another look at the world. I spent a year in Vietnam, going up and down the rivers of the Mekong Delta. Returning to UCSC in 1970 to complete my B.A. in psychology, I participated in a seminar studying the symbolism of labyrinths and helped build a large redwood labyrinth on the campus of the university. This project was like an alchemical opus because, once the labyrinth was completed, Baba Hari Dass, a silent yogi recently arrived from India, climbed up the spiral stairs to the top of the central tower and wrote on his little chalkboard: "I like this place." It was the beginning of the second primary subject of this

---

*Burckhardt, *Alchemy,* 87–88, 131–33.

book, my passionate study of ashtanga yoga, which has continued to this day.

In 1972, I set out to visit sacred sites across the United States, Europe, and North Africa. After visiting ancient stone circles, walled cities in Europe, and ancient Roman and Greek temples, I was eventually led to Crete, home of the famous mythological Minotaur and his labyrinth in Knossos. This turned out to be a perfect ending to my eastward journey. My next stop had been to visit the Great Pyramids of Giza, but alas, the 1973 Middle East war thwarted those plans. I traveled instead to the tiny Mediterranean island of Formentera, off the coast of Spain, and it was there, as Comet Kohoutek blazed overhead, that I began formulating some of the ideas in this book. While I was on Formentera at Christmastime in 1973, the rare occurrence of the comet's closest approach to Earth and the Sun—at the same time as a solar eclipse in Capricorn—inspired me to look forward to related astrological events. These events eventually included the great 1989–1990 alignment in Capricorn, the many grand crosses in the cardinal signs around 2010, and finally the Mayan Long Count end date of 2012, which was to end exactly on the winter solstice—and again Capricorn was accented.

Over time, experiencing and pondering these astrologically charged events proved helpful for putting together the pieces of this work, resulting in the Alchemical Tantric Arrangement with Capricorn as the final twelfth sign at the bottom of the astrological chart and Aquarius as the first sign. The major alignment of planets in Capricorn in 2020 was certainly another Hermetic milestone in this long journey of discovery.

The Alchemical Tantric Arrangement of the zodiac, like the Rosetta Stone, brings together three important systems: astrology, alchemy, and the chakra system of tantric yoga. Through this, we learn that embedded in the celestial wisdom of astrology are pointers toward a practical path to enlightenment. Clearly, the alchemists of old knew, or intuited, the importance of astrological timing and symbolism in their "royal art," and yoga masters to this day consider astrology a great boon on their path as well.

I am personally excited to continue my astrological studies with the help of this insightful perspective and to augment my yoga practice with the added element of astrological timing for auspicious alchemical and tantric cycles. I believe that there is fortunate synchronicity in the fact that a wonderful alignment of planets transited the potent Chiron portal between Capricorn and Aquarius in the years around 2020 and 2021, which included the publication of this book. I feel that I have been especially blessed in my life, and looking at my standard natal and Hermetic charts tends to substantiate this view.

And now for you folks, the readers, I truly hope that this book serves you on your path and is also fun and entertaining. Thank you for putting your trust in this undertaking, and I mean that in a truly Hermetic sense.

Love and Namaste,
Frederick Hamilton "Rico" Baker

Uncovering Astrology's Rosetta Stone

The primary purpose of this book is to present an innovative discovery, hidden in plain sight, that connects astrology and yoga, specifically the signs of the zodiac with the chakras of tantric yoga. Astrology, fundamentally, describes patterns in the changing world of phenomena and is highly dualistic. Yoga, ultimately, is about union and the clear recognition of nonduality. Hence, there is an underlying paradox—duality and nonduality. This vital paradox is woven throughout the book.

Important results of this discovery include the new perspectives given to the seven chakras by their association with planets and the twelve signs of the zodiac. This discovery creates a fundamental spiritual arrangement for astrology and opens up vast new horizons, including the possibility of a modern scientific understanding of what might be called miracles.

Inspired by modern feminism and the ancient goddess-oriented culture of Crete, as reflected in images used throughout this book, I am committed to gender balance in astrology. Although there has been considerable progress, modern astrology continues to rely on many classical Greek and Roman myths that denigrate the feminine.

In the later part of the book, I will explore the grand alignment that occurred in Capricorn in the year 2020 followed by the conjunction of

Jupiter and Saturn at the beginning of Aquarius. As will be demonstrated, this alignment was part of a series of related alignments featuring two signs highly accented in this book: Capricorn and Aquarius. What I am calling the 2020 vision is based on my research and intuition that the years surrounding 2020 would be particularly charged and would provide an excellent opportunity to make good use of the information in this book for a deeper understanding of astrology and for personal evolution.

Along the way, we'll discuss alchemy, the science and ethnobotany of DNA, archetypal psychology, numerology, sacred geometry, and the longer cycles of time. I will show you how you can add the insights of the Alchemical Tantric Arrangement to expand possibilities in astrology chart interpretation, and I will present meditations to connect you to these powerful forces in your mind and body.

The synthesis of these seemingly disparate traditions can provide a fresh perspective on the meanings within and can lead to a deeper understanding for beginning and advanced astrologers alike.

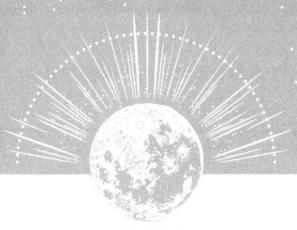

PART 1

✦✦✦

FUNDAMENTALS OF THREE SYMBOLIC SYSTEMS

Creating the Alchemical Tantric Arrangement

    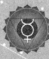

1
The Traditional Symbolism of Astrology and the Chakras

An easy way to introduce the amazing discovery of the surprising connections among astrology, alchemy, and the tantric yoga chakras, which form the basis for what will be described in this book as the Alchemical Tantric Arrangement (ATA), is to start with a diagram of the traditional zodiac. In Western astrology, the natural or basic arrangement of the twelve signs of the zodiac, along with their associated houses and ruling planets, is shown in figure 1.1. Notice the two signs, Cancer and Leo, ruled by the Moon and the Sun, in the lower right of the diagram. Moving upward, two signs, Gemini and Virgo, are both ruled by Mercury; moving up farther, two signs, Taurus and Libra, are both ruled by Venus. This order of dual rulership is continued upward through the planets Mars, Jupiter, and Saturn.

The key to understanding the Alchemical Tantric Arrangement (ATA) comes by rotating the natural zodiac so that the two signs ruled by Saturn—Capricorn and Aquarius—appear at the exact bottom of the wheel. From this slight alteration, surprising connections of symbolism across mythology, alchemy, tantric practices, and more are suddenly revealed. Like the Rosetta Stone, the ATA now allows us to use one language to discover new meanings in the others. To

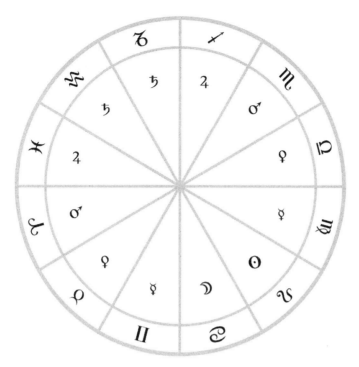

Fig. 1.1. The natural zodiac

understand and incorporate these amazing connections, we will further explore the meanings and mythology below.

THE SIGNS AND SYMBOLS OF ASTROLOGY

Astrology can be viewed as a storehouse packed with symbolism. A presentation of each sign of the zodiac, including its ruling planet, element, quality, number, gender, and image and more offers a deep, imaginal, poetic, and multifaceted vista. The following definitions are an introduction; more information about astrological concepts can be found in chapter 2.

Ruling Planet

Each sign of the zodiac has a planet or two (including dwarf planets and asteroids) that are particularly suited to the symbolism and essence of that sign. The traditional planetary rulership of the signs is a key to revealing a pattern based on the arrangement of alchemical elements, from lead in Capricorn and Aquarius to gold and silver in Leo and Cancer.

Quality

Three qualities or modes—cardinal, fixed, and mutable—also repeat around the zodiac. They follow a pattern: (1) an originating activity (cardinal), (2) a resulting structure (fixed), and (3) dissolution in preparation for a new activity (mutable). Aries, Cancer, Libra, and Capricorn are cardinal signs. Taurus, Leo, Scorpio, and Aquarius are fixed, and Gemini, Virgo, Sagittarius, and Pisces are the mutable signs.

Number

Each of the twelve numbers of the zodiac signs has a metaphysical, symbolic, geometrical, and mathematical connotation that colors the sign. Numerology is a vital part of astrology and yoga. Note that the natural zodiac is traditionally shown with the first sign, Aries, on the eastern, or left, side of the chart to follow the rising of the signs as viewed in the Northern Hemisphere. The twelve houses follow this counterclockwise numbering. However, the numbering of signs and houses in the Alchemical Tantric Arrangement system starts with Aquarius at the bottom of the astrological chart, an arrangement that is further explained in chapter 2. (See also chapter 8 for more on astrological numerology.)

Element, Gender, and Age

There are four traditional elements that repeat themselves around the circle of the zodiac: fire, earth, air, and water, which correspond in astrology, respectively, to active, grounded, intellectual, and emotional. Another arrangement—earth, water, air, and fire—corresponds to solid, liquid, gas, and plasma, the four states of matter.

Earth and water elements have a traditional symbolic connection to the receptive and feminine, while fire and air are associated with the active and masculine. The three members of each of the four elements can further be meaningfully divided into youth, adult, and elder, which adds an extra measure of meaning to the twelve signs.

GENDER AND AGE ATTRIBUTES OF THE SIGNS

ELEMENT	GENDER	YOUTH	ADULT	ELDER
Earth	Feminine	Virgo	Taurus	Capricorn
Water	Feminine	Scorpio	Cancer	Pisces
Fire	Masculine	Aries	Leo	Sagittarius
Air	Masculine	Gemini	Libra	Aquarius

Animal or Zodiac Image and Direction

The animals or other images that represent each sign of the zodiac carry a symbolic set of associations that convey great depth of meaning.

The natural zodiac is placed around a circle representing, in two dimensions, a view of the path of the planets, with Aries on the left or east. Thus, the symbolism of the four directions (north, east, south, west) is included in the signs of the natural zodiac: the four cardinal and mutable signs share the four cardinal directions. The four cross-quarter times of the year, known as the four seasonal holidays of Beltain, Lamas, Halloween, and Candlemas, fall into the midpoints of the four fixed signs. The direction of each sign is based on this scheme.

Body Part, Color, and Holidays

Starting with Aries at the head and proceeding down through the human body to Pisces at the feet, each sign has an associated body part that adds to its overall meaning. Each sign has an associated color or colors that adds to the overall feeling tone. The holidays celebrated during each sign of the zodiac are revealing symbolically.

THE SYMBOLISM OF THE CHAKRAS

Although an in-depth study of the chakras of tantric yoga could be a lifelong project, here I simply want to develop their symbolism further for better understanding of how they relate to the astrological signs. The chakras are an integral part of Tantra, the ancient occult wisdom of India. Himalayan yogi Baba Hari Dass has said that Tantra predates the Vedas, so Tantra is similar to other ancient traditions like those that produced the I Ching, astrology, alchemy, Kabbalah, and the lineage of Thoth/Hermes.

The Sanskrit word *chakra* means "wheel," and the chakras can be envisioned as spinning wheels of energy. Traditionally, there are seven chakras, each with a Sanskrit name that suggests its esoteric meaning.

First chakra—*Muladhara,* meaning "root support"
Second chakra—*Svadisthana,* meaning "self-dwelling"
Third chakra—*Manipura,* meaning "jeweled city"
Fourth chakra—*Anahata,* meaning "unstruck sound"
Fifth chakra—*Vishuddha,* meaning "purification"
Sixth chakra—*Ajna,* meaning "command"
Seventh chakra—*Sahasrara,* meaning "thousand petals"

In addition to the Sanskrit names, there are several metaphors that have been commonly used to lend meaning to the chakra system including: the human body, the elements, the tree, and, perhaps especially in California, the automobile. Various commentators have written about the chakras from many perspectives, including the Swiss psychiatrist and psychoanalyst Carl G. Jung, who makes a comparison of the chakras to his concepts of the psyche. Other psychologists have noted the similarities with theories of psychological development. At the other end of the spectrum, many consider the chakras to be a primarily physical phenomenon and correlated with nerves and endocrine glands. Between these extremes of psyche and soma, the chakras are seen as wheels of energy, or vortexes, in the subtle body. The chakras are clearly images rich with meaning.

The human body is a common way to portray the symbolism of the chakras. Human physiology can be associated with the chakras—for example, the nervous, circulatory, hormonal, lymph systems, and so on.

The subtle elements, earth, water, fire, air, and ether, and the super-subtle elements, sound and light, also contribute to the meaning of the seven chakras.

Earth contributes a grounded, materialistic quality to the first chakra.

Water suggests a flowing emotional quality to the second chakra.

Fire suggests heat and is connected to the digestive fire of the third chakra.

Air with its motion is connected to the changeable feelings of the fourth chakra.

Ether symbolizes the spaciousness of mind and communication of the fifth chakra.

Sound vibrates with the creativity of the sixth chakra.

Light corresponds with the radiance of life and unconditional love of the seventh chakra.

When the symbolism of the human body is combined with the subtle elements, we see a progression: from the urgency of earthy defecation related to the first chakra, to watery urination of the second chakra, and the urgency of hunger to feed the fires of digestion to maintain our 98.6 degrees in the third chakra. Ascending the chakras, the elements become subtler, and the literal urgency decreases. The airy fourth chakra seems to relate to the need for touch, relationship, and intimacy. The fifth chakra, related to the subtle element of ether, or space, can be associated with the need to communicate; the sixth chakra is related to the higher mind, while the seventh chakra can be linked with the subtle need for union with the Ultimate.

Following is another, related way of describing the psychological progression:

The first chakra is about survival.

The second chakra is about reproduction.

The third chakra is about the will to power.

The fourth chakra is about the need for social connection.
The fifth chakra is about the importance of communication.
The sixth chakra is about developing the higher mind.
The seventh chakra is about transcendence.

Trees, in general, but specifically the World Tree, or Tree of Life, provide a rich metaphor when applied to the seven chakras.

The first, or root, chakra, like the roots of the tree, provides support and earthy elemental nurturance.

The second, or sacral, chakra is like the sap or a sacred liquid essence carrying food upward through the trunk.

The third, or navel, chakra is like the protective bark that protects the tree from outside threats.

The fourth, or heart, chakra is similar to the central heartwood.

The fifth, or throat, chakra, like the major branches of the tree, represents the transition into the air and ether elements.

The sixth, or brow, chakra suggests the movement of leaves, singing in the breeze.

The seventh, or crown, chakra communicates with the solar light from above.

The *automobile* (a word meaning "self-mobile" or "mobile self") is another suggestive metaphor to portray the workings of the seven chakras. The first chakra, like the gas tank, contributes energy to operate the second chakra, which, like a generator, supplies the electrical charge to fire the cylinders of the third chakra, giving power to turn the four wheels of the fourth chakra, guided by the steering wheel of the fifth chakra and the headlights of the sixth and seventh chakras.

CHAKRAS AND THE ZODIAC

In the tantric system, each chakra is represented by a lotus blossom and is associated with a specific mantra. In the Alchemical Tantric

Arrangement system, the chakras are further aligned with the astrological signs and their ruling planets, plus related stars and constellations.

Capricorn and Aquarius (Saturn and Uranus) are aligned with the first root chakra.

Sagittarius and Pisces (Jupiter and Neptune) are aligned with the second sacral chakra.

Scorpio and Aries (Pluto and Mars) are aligned with the third navel chakra.

Libra and Taurus (Venus) are aligned with the fourth heart chakra.

Virgo and Gemini (Mercury) are aligned with the fifth throat chakra.

Cancer (and Moon) are aligned with the sixth brow or third eye chakra.

Leo (and Sun) are aligned with the seventh crown chakra.

The relationships between the chakras and the signs are explored in depth in chapter 5, but what follows are the essential symbolic associations. Please note that in general I follow the chakra symbolism taken from the *Ashtanga Yoga Primer* by Baba Hari Dass; however, with the following chakras I have exclusively used the progression of the seven colors of the rainbow, which diverge in several cases from the *Primer*.

The first chakra, or Muladhara, symbolized by a red four-petaled lotus with a golden square, is related to the base of the spine, the tailbone, and the anus, giving it a humble but important connection to the bottom, the seat, and elimination. This chakra is connected with Saturn and Uranus, the associated planets, and with the signs and constellations of Capricorn and Aquarius.

Earth is the element of the first chakra, and its mantra is *lang*. The star at the beginning of the sign Aquarius is Altair, in the constellation of the Eagle. In myth, this eagle belongs to Zeus, and it was in this form that the king of the gods grabbed the beautiful boy Ganymede and carried him up to Olympus to be the cupbearer to the divinities.

The second chakra, or Svadisthana, symbolized by an orange six-petaled lotus with a crescent Moon, is related to the area of the body at the sacrum and genitals. It carries the highly charged, sacred, and hard-wired assignment of pleasure and sexual reproduction and is a powerful generator of energy. It is also connected to urination. Jupiter and Neptune are associated with this chakra, as are the signs and constellations of Sagittarius and Pisces. Water is the element of the second chakra, and its mantra is *vang*. The Galactic Center, the center of our Milky Way Galaxy, is located in the sign and constellation of Sagittarius.

The third chakra, or Manipura, a yellow ten-petaled lotus with a fiery red triangle as symbol, is related to the area of the navel, the stomach and intestines, and also the adrenal glands. It carries rich symbolic associations with our primal connection to the mother, the womb, the belly, deep nurturance, the fire of digestion, and power. This chakra is connected to Mars and Pluto and the signs and constellations of Scorpio and Aries. An important bright star in Scorpio is Antares. Fire is the element of the third chakra, and its mantra is *rang*.

The fourth chakra, or Anahata, a green twelve-petaled lotus with a green six-pointed star, is related to the heart and the solar plexus, giving it associations with love and centrality. Venus, the traditional ruler of Libra and Taurus, is connected to this chakra. Eris, a dwarf planet discovered in 2005, I tentatively consider as a ruler of these signs and connected to the fourth chakra. The Libra constellation has two bright stars in the form of an archway, according to Vedic astrology, or what I like to imagine as a "stargate." These stars were formerly seen as the two pincers of the neighboring Scorpion but now are seen as the two pans of the balance. The Taurus constellation contains the bright star Aldebaran, also called the Eye of the Bull. Air is the element of the fourth chakra, and its mantra is *yang*.

The fifth chakra, or Vishuddha, a blue sixteen-petaled lotus with a sparkling blue or white circle as symbol, is related to the throat, neck, and thyroid, associating it with speech and being the connector between the head and the lower body. Space, or ether, is the element, and the mantra is *hang*. The planet Mercury, the Virgo constellation with her bright star Spica, and the Gemini constellation with the twin stars Castor and Pollux are all connected to this chakra.

The sixth chakra, or Ajna, a blue-violet two-petaled lotus with a silver lunar crescent, is related to the brow, the prefrontal cortex, and the pineal gland. As such, it is linked with higher functions of the mind, including insight and intuition. This chakra is related to the super-subtle element of sound, and its mantra is *thang,* like the ringing of a bell in the skull.

The seventh chakra, or Sahasrara, a multipetaled multicolored lotus with the golden Sun as a symbol, is related to the top of the head, crown, and skull. It thereby carries the symbolic quality of knowledge beyond or transcendent of human limitations. The Sun and the constellation of Leo with its bright royal star Regulus are connected to this chakra. (Due to precession, Regulus has now moved into the sign of Virgo, which is important because it correlates with more and more emphasis on the empowerment of women.) The crown chakra is related to the super-subtle element of light and the mantra of *om,* or *aum.*

These are the fundamentals of two of the three systems. Perhaps you can already see some of the powerful correlations we'll explore as we build the Alchemical Tantric Arrangement.

2
Journey through the Twelvefold Signs

We shall now set out on a pilgrimage through the rich symbolism of the twelve signs of the zodiac, emphasizing the added meaning gained through the association with the tantric yoga chakras. The astrological, mythological, and numerological aspects of each sign are explored in depth. Included in the description of each sign is the alchemical metal with which it is associated. (We explore the alchemical aspect of each sign later in chapter 4.)

A WORD
ABOUT MYTHOLOGY

Myth is an integral part of daily life, in the form of the stories we live by, which is the subject of archetypal psychology. It is a vital part of astrology and yoga, and in this chapter there is an emphasis on the mythological aspects of the signs.

But it is important to note the politics involved in myth, especially the *his*-torical shift to patriarchal values, which negatively affected the way goddesses and women were portrayed. Whenever a myth portrays a goddess in a demeaning way, it is likely that a political agenda is involved. It is for this reason that I greatly appreciate the scholarship of Jane Ellen Harrison, who highlighted this phenomenon in her writings on mythology. In the sign descriptions that follow, I have attempted to point out where a patriarchal society has adversely affected and modified earlier matriarchal myths.

I am also sensitive to the fact that mythology is a huge, complex subject. In this book I do not have the space to give an in-depth treatment of all the myths related to the planets and constellations. My astronomer friend, professor John Stocke, Ph.D., is writing a book he has been sharing with me on the constellations of different cultures; I hope it will be widely available. Another brilliant book that I especially enjoy about myth, recommended by James Hillman, is *Gods of the Greeks* by Károly Kerényi. It should be noted that, although there is much equivalence between Greek and Roman myths—for example, Zeus and Jupiter are both the king of the gods—there are also major differences between the two.

A TURN OF
THE ZODIAC WHEEL

The new Alchemical Tantric Arrangement (ATA) is created by a simple, yet profound, rotation of the natural zodiac that places Cancer and Leo at the top of the wheel and Capricorn and Aquarius at the bottom, revealing a radically new (and also ancient) arrangement. (See Plate 1 for a full illustration.) The order of the signs is the same; however, the ATA now begins with Aquarius, rather than Aries, as the first sign, and starts at the bottom of the chart rather than the left side, which allows a highly symbolic order of the planets to appear. We'll explore the reasons for this change and the meanings it can reveal in chapter 4. But for now, we begin our in-depth exploration of the mythology and symbolism surrounding the zodiac with the first sign in the ATA.

AQUARIUS

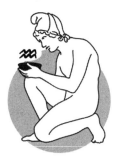

Ruling planet: Uranus (and Saturn)

Associated asteroid: Chiron

Also associated: Ketu, the Moon's south node, or the tail of the dragon

Element: Air

Quality: Fixed

Numbers: Natural zodiac 11, Hermetic 1

Relative age: Elder

Gender: Masculine

Zodiac image: Cupbearer, angel

Body part: Ankles

Direction: Southeast

Colors: Clear, sky blue

Alchemical metal: Uranium (and lead)

Holidays: Imbolc/Candlemas, Brigid's Day, Groundhog Day, St. Valentine's Day, Freedom Day, President's Day, Chinese New Year. (The month of February comes from the Latin time of purification. February is unusual, having only twenty-eight days, or twenty-nine days in leap years.)

Mythology: Ganymede, Apollo, Daedalus and Icarus, Prometheus, Hebe, Saturn, Ouranus, Adam and Eve and the serpent, Ketu/the dragon's tail (lord of the south lunar node), Chiron

Chakra: First, Muladhara (root support), base of the spine, anus
Symbol: Red four-petaled lotus containing a golden square or cube

Mantra: *Lang*

Element: Earth

Concerns: Food, resources, survival, safety, security, material, physical life

Planets: Saturn and Uranus, also Chiron and the south node of the Moon

Fig. 2.1. First, or root, chakra, Muladhara

Aquarian Astrology

The sign Aquarius is often referred to as the Water Bearer because it is depicted as a person pouring liquid out of a vessel. However, rather than simply water, it is the "ambrosia of immortality" that is contained in the vessel, and it is being poured out to all the divinities on Mount Olympus. The womb-shaped vessel is like the alchemical alembic, and the ambrosia is like the *ojas,* or tantric spiritual fluid.

In classical Greek mythology, the cupbearer was Ganymede, who was Zeus's handsome young lover, suggesting tantric rather than reproductive union. In earlier Greek myth, there was a goddess who was the bearer of immortality, Hebe, a virgin form of the Great Mother Goddess. She was the keeper of the Tree of Life, whose magic apples imparted immortality to the divinities. This tree was guarded by Hebe's personal serpent. This is a very different serpent story from the one featuring Adam and Eve. Nevertheless, the Tree of Life and the serpent are certainly reminiscent of the kundalini serpent wrapped around the tantric lingam at the base of the spine and the "tree" of the chakras.

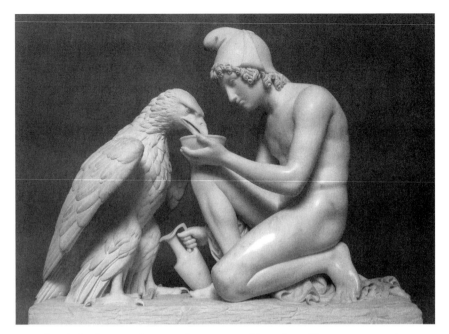

Fig. 2.2. Ganymede provides a cup of liquid to Zeus, as an eagle.
Granymede Waters Zeus as an Eagle by Bertel Thorvaldsen, 1817.
Thorvaldsen Museum, Copenhagen.

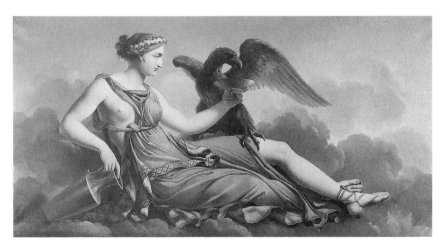

Fig. 2.3. Hebe offers a cup to her father, Zeus, embodied as an eagle.
Hebe by Jacques Louis Dubois, 1810.

Aquarius is a fixed air sign, and hence the liquid the cupbearer pours
out is the heavenly ambrosia of knowledge and wisdom. The air signs

are associated with the intellect, and the fixed signs contain the powerful cross-quarter times of the year. The midpoint of Aquarius corresponds to the subtle beginnings of spring in the Northern Hemisphere, considered by some cultures, such as the Chinese, to be the beginning of the year. The first stirrings of spring emphasize the increasing light.

Aquarius is the first sign of the Hermetic arrangement and the eleventh sign of the natural zodiac, 1 and 1 repeated. Eleven is a master number, and 1 is a perfect number to begin the upward, accumulating path. Indeed, Aquarius pours out heavenly information and is a sign related to spiritual mastery. The traditional ruler of this sign was Saturn, and the new ruler is Uranus, considered to have associations with Prometheus, bringer of light and fire to humanity. Aquarius carries many of the same qualities as its ruling planet, Uranus: humanitarian, idealistic, innovative, unique, inventive, radical, and rebellious.

Brilliant Apollo is another archetype related to Aquarius: his light is bright, but he casts a big shadow. Although Aquarius is indeed radiant, folks with this Sun sign can think that they are favored with divine right, like Apollo, who felt that he was the especially honored carrier of his father Zeus's knowledge.

Mercury is exalted in the sign of Aquarius, and there is a revealing story of the rivalry between Apollo, the older brother, and Hermes, the baby brother. Immediately after his birth, Hermes stole Apollo's cattle, and father Zeus had to intervene. Hermes (Mercury to the Romans) has a special connection to Aquarius via his caduceus, or talking stick, which is similar in shape to the tantric yoga chakra system, both having a central rod and two intertwining serpents.

The Aquarian Age is popularly known as the New Age, when we are starting anew. It is often related to the positive qualities of humanitarian values and brilliant scientific and technological advancements. However, every sign has its up side and down side, and Aquarius is no exception. Like its association with uranium and the age of nuclear power and radioactivity, Aquarius also carries the shadow side of science and technology, where our seemingly clever inventions often return to haunt us, like Dr. Frankenstein's monster.

In terms of the Alchemical Tantric Arrangement, Aquarius holds the duality of both conservative Saturn and innovative Uranus. The cusp at the beginning of Aquarius therefore functions as an important portal that I call the portal of Chiron (see more about this portal in chapter 7). This portal symbolizes either continuing on the wheel of the zodiac, with the *ida* and *pingala nadis,* or turning inward toward the central *sushumna nadi* and the awakening of kundalini (see more about the nadis in chapter 3).

Aquarian Mythology

Uranus and Saturn

There is an interesting twist to the dynamic between Saturn, the son, and Uranus, the father, for it appears in astrology that Saturn, the son, is the conservative limiter, while Uranus, the father, is the wild innovator, acting more like a rebellious Prometheus. Apparently, Uranus, after his separation from Gaia, started to get wildly creative. In astrology, Uranus has become the planet of the New Age and also the new planet of both astrology and technology. Considering that uranium is the alchemical metal for Uranus, we can see another connection to Prometheus the Titan, who gave fire to humans and received harsh punishment from Zeus for doing so. The modern radioactive fire of atomic energy is another dubious "gift" that seems to have come with dire consequences. A burning question for the Aquarian Age will be whether we can survive this powerful gift of technology and all of the more potent and problematic Aquarian "gifts" that are already coming our way in what might be called a perfect storm of technology. See Richard Tarnas's brilliant *Prometheus The Awakener* for a discussion of Prometheus and Uranus.

Chiron

Chiron, called the wounded healer, is an asteroid located between the orbits of Saturn and Uranus. Chiron's glyph looks like a key, and indeed its healing energy is key to opening the way to spiritual evolution. Chiron offers great promise that we can heal our traumas (perhaps

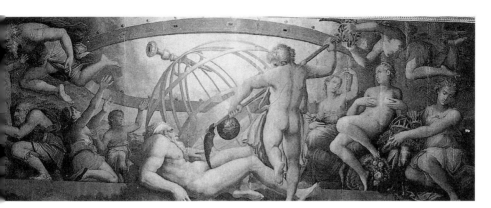

Fig. 2.4. Saturn/Cronus separating the primal unity of Uranus and Gaia.
The Mutilation of Uranus by Saturn by Giorgio Vasari and Gherardi Christofano,
1554–1556.

related to deeply hidden patterns) and can learn from these experiences, thereby becoming a seasoned healer for others with similar challenges.

Chiron, the centaur of Greek myth, was the son of Cronus (Saturn to the Romans) in his horse form. He became known for kindness, wisdom, and justice. He was the teacher of many Greek heroes. He was skilled in archery, healing, and the medicinal uses of wild plants, which he learned from the goddess Artemis, also a skilled archer. Chiron is credited with being the teacher of Asclepius, the archetypal physician. It is also notable that Chiron was considered to be a great astrologer.

As a centaur, Chiron represents integrating the human and animal parts of the psyche and hence integration in general. Chiron was a universal teacher, especially of youth, and taught a wide variety of subjects to his students.

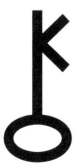

Fig. 2.5. The symbol
of Chiron

Although Chiron is also related to the sign Sagittarius the centaur, in the Alchemical Tantric Arrangement of the zodiac, Chiron is an important gatekeeper at the cusp between Capricorn, ruled by Saturn, and Aquarius, ruled by Uranus. Hence, Chiron watches over the pivotal point in the transition from the traditional visible planets to the outer planets and from the traditional seven alchemical metals to the radioactive alchemical metals. It is the place where kundalini energy can be awakened, opening to the central path upward through the chakras. Chiron's curved bow and straight arrow represent the meeting of the curve of the zodiac signs with the straight central axis of the chakras, leading to profound awakening.

Rahu and Ketu

Rahu and Ketu have a mythological story that has some similarities to Prometheus in that they were created when they were in the form of a demon who was stealing ambrosia from the gods. The larger story, called "Churning the Ocean of Milk," says that the god Vishnu had assumed the form of a gigantic turtle on whose back the central pillar of Mt. Meru was being rotated by the gods and demons. They were tugging on either end of a huge serpent, which caused the ocean of milk to churn. Many wonderful objects were churned out of this milky sea, including the ambrosia of immortality. The ambrosia thereby produced was then distributed only to the gods until one of the demons jumped in and took a drink, making him immortal. Vishnu, not appreciating this action, cut the serpent demon, now immortal, in two with his discus, creating an immortal head and tail, or Rahu and Ketu.

The points on the zodiac represented by Rahu and Ketu correspond to the highly charged times of solar and lunar eclipses, when it is said that the demons temporarily swallow the Sun and/or Moon. Also called the head and tail of the dragon, these so-called shadow planets have resonance with Uranus and hence Prometheus. As dragons or serpents, they are appropriately placed in this first chakra along with the serpent of awakening named Kundalini. Rahu and Ketu have a shadowy trickster side in Vedic astrology, as does the serpent of Adam and Eve fame.

John Major Jenkins, in his book *Galactic Alignment,* presents this story of Rahu and Ketu, the Moon's nodes, and their considerable connections with the precession of the equinoxes and solstices and the 2012 era alignment with the galactic equator. The nodes, like the movement of precession, move primarily in a retrograde direction, or opposite to the forward motion of the planets. This retrograde motion, in astrology, suggests that we stop, take a closer look, and re-view the situation because something unusual and important is happening.

Aquarius's path of awakening and potential immortality is apparently fraught with danger and is something that brings resistance from the heavenly beings. Could this be a reference to the Anunnaki, a group of powerful ancient Middle Eastern deities/E.T.s? A psychological way of saying this is that humans have a preprogrammed resistance to moving from the mortal human to the immortal divine. Aquarius is associated with the root chakra, and this chakra's powerful potential for awakening is why the ambivalent image of the serpent or dragon is involved.

Hopefully, the world learned a great deal more about Aquarius and its highly charged potential after Jupiter and Saturn came together at the beginning of this sign at the end of 2020. Pluto, divinity of the apocalypse, will also enter Aquarius in 2023. This time period, as many planets transition into Aquarius, will give us some good hints concerning the meaning of the New Age of Aquarius.

PISCES

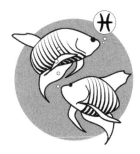

Ruling planet: Neptune (and Jupiter)
Associated asteroid or dwarf planet: Salacia
Element: Water
Quality: Mutable
Numbers: Natural zodiac 12, Hermetic 2
Relative age: Elder
Gender: Feminine
Zodiac image: Two fish
Body part: Feet
Direction: East
Color: Sea blue-green
Alchemical metal: Neptunium (and tin)
Holidays: Purim, International Women's Day, St. Patrick's Day
Mythology: Neptune/Poseidon, Salacia/Amphitrite, Hecate, Vishnu, Jupiter/Zeus
Chakra: Second, Svadisthana (one's own base), sacral, genital center
   Symbol: Orange six-petaled lotus
   Mantra: *Vang*
   Element: Water, represented by the silver crescent Moon
   Concerns: Pleasure, sexuality, vital force, unconscious emotions and desires
   Planets: Jupiter, Neptune

Piscean Astrology

The sensitive sign of Pisces is a mutable water sign, which makes it exceptionally changeable and, like water, able to flow into almost any

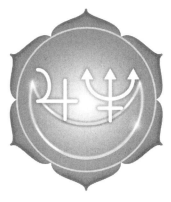

Fig. 2.6. Second, or sacral, chakra, Svadisthana

container. Pisces is known for its limitless ability to "go with the flow." As the twelfth and final sign in the natural zodiac, it is the repository of all the patterns of all the cycles, like the great sea, which receives water from all the rivers and directly from heavenly rain. Twelve is the defining number of astrology and is the basis of astrology's ability to integrate so much diversity. The number 12 is able to be divided by the numbers 1, 2, 3, 4, 6, and 12 and is rich with associations, as in the twelve disciples, twelve tribes of Israel, twelve jurors, twelve months, twelve daylight hours, etc.

Pisces is represented by two yin-yang fish, seemingly swimming in opposite directions; however, in fact, both are part of the great circular whole and are often shown connected by a cord. Pisces is extremely sensitive and is often in touch with other worlds and dimensions, the basis for what are often called Pisces's psychic abilities. These psychic abilities make perfect sense when we recall that Pisces, like the ocean, represents totality, so it is no wonder that this sign is in communication with realms beyond normal third-dimensional reach.

Being limitless and without boundaries, it is often difficult for a Pisces person to function in consensus reality, and she or he may appear at times to be spacey or drifty. They may appear to be out of touch because they are in touch with such large realms. This sign tends to embody compassion, and again, this makes sense when we consider that Pisceans are living in an oceanic world where everything is indeed highly interconnected.

Because Pisces folks often lack strong boundaries and are compassionate, passive, and caring toward others, they are likely to overextend their energy. This can result in burnout or perhaps better stated as washout and may also result in the gentle fish becoming an aggressive shark. Persons with Pisces accented in their natal chart are being strongly affected at this time by Neptune, the ruling planet of Pisces, moving through this deep oceanic sign of the fishes.

Piscean Mythology

Salacia

The mythology of the sign of the fishes is as rich as the sea, teeming with watery life. Of course, life itself is highly dependent on water, and this is reflected in the images of the great ocean goddesses like Salacia and Amphitrite and their partners, Neptune and Poseidon. On September 22, 2004, three American astronomers discovered a relatively large minor planet, which was later named Salacia, along with its only moon, which was named Actaea. Salacia has an orbit with a duration of 271 years, close to that of Pluto, but with a very different inclination. On its discovery date, Salacia was appropriately in the sign of Pisces. Presently, she is at the beginning of Aries, and this placement could very easily be viewed as associated with the intense sexual drama of these times (for example, the scandals surrounding the late Jeffrey Epstein).

Salacia (called Amphitrite in Greek mythology) was the partner and queen of the sea with Neptune in Roman myth and is said to have hidden from Neptune until a dolphin found her. Neptune rewarded the dolphin by placing its image in the stars as the constellation Delphinus. Although Salacia has been connected to the spicy word *salacious,* in her mythology she would appear to be quite shy. Her etymology is also related to the word *salt,* as in saltwater. It is appropriate to place Salacia with Neptune in the watery and sexual second chakra. Together, they created innumerable offspring, and so regarding reproduction, they were definitely active.

Poseidon and Ancient Crete

On the island queendom of ancient Crete, myth tells of Poseidon, Greek god of the sea, coming ashore dramatically out of the waves in the form of a beautiful white bull with golden horns. Poseidon was known on Crete in the powerful forms of both horse and bull. He was the earth shaker, and his roar and rumble were known on the island as the terrifying approach of an earthquake and tsunami.

The gender-balanced culture of ancient Crete was one of the most artistic and peaceful in the Mediterranean region until the invasion by the warrior cultures of the north. The myths produced by later patriarchal Greek culture demonstrate their negativity toward the feminine. Such misogyny is present in their strange story of the Cretan Minotaur, which tells of Queen Pasiphaë mating with the Bull from the Sea (Poseidon) to create the monstrous Minotaur, which was later imprisoned in the labyrinth. Actually, on ancient Crete, the Great Goddess was supreme, the queen was her servant, and the labyrinth was the vast royal temple or palace of Knossos, designed by the architect and inventor Daedalus, probably with plenty of help from joyously artistic men and women. King Minos, son of Zeus and king of Crete, wore the bull mask, and Ariadne knew how to thread her way through the labyrinth and to dance the bull dance because she was its royal princess. For these qualities, I chose an artistic depiction of Ariadne to be the central figure of the Alchemical Tantric Arrangement throughout this book.

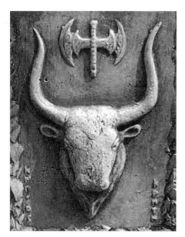

Fig. 2.7. Bull and labrys, Palace of Knossos, Heraklion, Crete, 1100 BCE.

Fig. 2.8.
Medallion from
ancient Crete.
Note the Sun
and Moon,
labrys, fruit,
poppies, and
dresses.

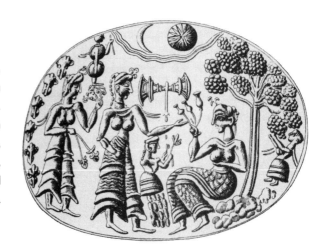

Fig. 2.9. The labrys,
the double-headed ax,
a symbol of the Great
Goddess

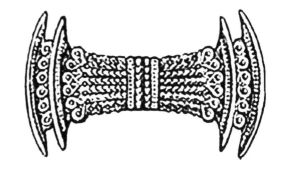

The word *labyrinth* originates in *labrys*, the Lydian word for the double-headed ax. Like the cow, the ax was a powerful symbol of the goddess and is also perhaps a gender-balanced symbol. In keeping with Pisces's association with the second chakra, the double-headed ax head can represent the vulva and the ax's handle the phallus. The young women and men of Crete deeply respected and honored the power of Poseidon, god of the sea, so much so that they danced through the great bull's horns and vaulted over his back. They played in awe with their mighty god. An archaeologist named the ancient civilization of Crete "Minoan" after King Minos, a legendary figure out of Greek mythology; however, it is questionable whether the Minoans followed a powerful king rather than a more gender-balanced leadership.

Hecate

Hecate is known as the great-grandmother or crone. She was once the goddess ruler of the three realms—Earth, Ocean, and Underworld—and now shares these realms with her Olympian brothers. In the stories of Hades (Roman Pluto) and Persephone (Roman Proserpina), Hecate was the observer of the stealing of Persephone by Hades and reported this to Helios, who then told Zeus (Roman Jupiter), who convinced his underworldly brother, Hades, to release Persephone for half of each year. Hecate resonates with Pisces and Neptune since they are associated with the all-embracing sea that welcomes all the rivers into its wide womb. Pisces and the twelfth house are the final sign and house of the natural zodiac and, as such, are rich with experience and are like the womb that gives birth to the continuing cycles of life.

Vishnu

Vishnu is the blue-colored Hindu divinity of preservation, often pictured floating in the great primal sea on the back of a huge serpent. He has taken on many forms called avatars over vast periods of time. Each avatar comes when needed to restore balance to the deteriorating world. His forms as Rama and Krishna are perhaps the most well known, although his forms as fish and turtle are certainly fitting for Pisces. We need to be especially aware of Vishnu's presence in these challenging and chaotic times. Since we are supposedly in a dark age now, we may be feeling an especially strong pull of these two opposing directions, the spiritual and the material, accenting the image of the two fish swimming in opposite directions.

Jupiter/Zeus

Jupiter/Zeus is described as coming in many forms—such as a bull, swan, eagle, and shower of gold—and as mating with various goddesses and mortals. Although Jupiter is the traditional planet associated with the sign Pisces, and Neptune is the new ruling planet, both divine brothers are powerful images of fertile masculinity and have a resonance with the sexual water element of the second chakra.

ARIES

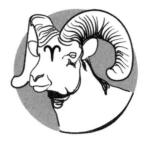

Ruling planet: Mars (and Pluto)
Associated asteroids: Pallas, Vesta
Element: Fire
Quality: Cardinal
Numbers: Natural zodiac 1, Hermetic 3
Relative age: Youth
Gender: Masculine
Zodiac image: Ram or sheep
Body part: Head
Direction: East
Color: Red
Alchemical metal: Iron
Holidays: Easter, Passover, Income Tax Day
Mythology: Mars/Ares, Golden Ram, Amazons, Pallas Athene, Easter, Pele
Chakra: Third, Manipura (jeweled city), navel, solar plexis
  Symbol: Yellow ten-petaled lotus with a fiery red triangle
  Mantra: *Rang*
  Element: Fire
  Planets: Mars and Pluto
  Concerns: Power, control, will, strength, focus

Arian Astrology

Although Aries is associated with the third chakra in the ATA, traditionally this is the first sign of the natural zodiac. It represents the

Fig. 2.10. Third, or navel, chakra, Manipura

power and drive of the number 1 and carries a flavor of midspring bursting forth into full flower. Aries is ruled by the fiery red planet, Mars, which emphasizes dynamic outgoing energy. Aries is a fire sign, and being in the cardinal direction of the great eastern Sun portrays the time of dawn and bursting forth of the light. Aries rules the head, and like the image of the ram with its great battering horns, the sign conveys headstrong drive and forceful strength. Aries can expect to experience blows to the head and accidents in general due to taking risks and engaging in reckless activities. Many Arians die young.

Arian Mythology

The Roman/Greek god Mars/Ares and goddess Minerva/Athena, the Golden Ram and Golden Fleece from Greek mythology, the Hawaiian Goddess Pele, and the Amazons all present mythological themes that shed light on the sign Aries.

Mars/Ares

Mars/Ares, as the god of war, is portrayed in myth as easily lost in the turmoil of battle and not necessarily a good strategist, in contrast to Athena, who was able to work out rational plans in the midst of battle. The Amazons are examples in myth of fierce female warriors. They were known as being skilled with horses, which gave them an advantage in battle. They were also said to defend their female-controlled territory from domination by the patriarchal warrior hordes. The Amazons are said to be descendants of Ares. They worshipped both Ares and Artemis.

Mars/Ares was portrayed as very handsome and attractive in the supermasculine sense. Lovely Venus/Aphrodite—although married to the lame metalworker of the fiery furnace, Vulcan/Hephaestus—had a passionate affair with Mars/Ares, and they conceived a child together named Concordia/Harmonia, perhaps as an expression of the balance of their two divergent characters.

The Golden Fleece

The Golden Fleece is a mythological theme related to both Ares and his totem animal, the ram. In one story, the Golden Ram was sacrificed to Zeus, and its fleece was placed in the temple of Ares, protected by a fiery dragon. Jason and the Argonauts went in search of and found the Golden Fleece, as did Hercules. The Golden Fleece is a symbol of authority and kingship.

Pele

Pele is the Hawaiian fire and volcano goddess who is credited with creating the Hawaiian Islands. She is known for her great power, passion, and for shape-shifting.

Oestre: An Aries Goddess

The Saxon goddess Oestre, whose name was given to the sacrificial festival later called Ostara, or Easter, is associated with the Moon hare, or Easter bunny. Her golden world egg is like that of Hathor in Egypt and Astarte in the Middle East; sometimes the egg was red or multicolored. The Moon is comparable to an oval egg or ovum and is likewise a fertility symbol. *Estrus,* or *oestrus,* is a similar word meaning "passionate frenzy" and is the period of ovulation during the fertility cycle. Easter is celebrated the Sunday after the full Moon following the spring equinox. The full Moon is like an ovum floating in amniotic fluid that has many flecks of matter, like stars. The many stars in the heavens represent the many souls that the goddess O-star-a or A-star-te is birthing into being.

Easter (and the name Esther) are related to asters or stars, which suggests a connection to astrology and the astral body.

Easter is also considered a goddess of the dawn and of the east, like Aries, the sign on the eastern horizon or ascendant. Aries, as the first sign of the new astrological year in the natural zodiac, is connected to rebirth and the ascendancy of the light principle. Aries is a time of spring and springing forth into action. It is a sign of activation, with sexual vigor abounding. It is a time of ejaculation and ovulation, resulting in fertilization associated with the next sign, Taurus. The sign before Aries, Pisces, can be seen as the rich and ripe time of full ovaries and testes, awaiting the time for their contents to spring forth.

Pluto/Hades and Radioactive Fire

Aries radiates its electromagnetic energy through the lens of the most cardinal of the fire signs. Cardinal means purest representative of its kind, and Aries is pure fire energy. "How and where is this fiery energy directed?" is the question; Aries is the will (sometimes with awareness lacking). Mighty Mars is the ruling planet of Aries, and fire is his element. Although Pluto is primarily associated with the sign Scorpio, due to the dual rulership of the third chakra, Pluto is also connected to Aries. Mars and Pluto are a resonant match for the fiery third chakra.

Pluto, as divinity of the apocalypse and the underworld, adds another level of depth and intensity to the story. Pluto's alchemical metal, plutonium, ushered in the age of radioactive nuclear fire. Like pouring gasoline on the fire, Pluto raises Mars's heat to overwhelming levels of magnitude. It is very interesting to realize how the trans-Saturnian planets (Uranus, Neptune, and Pluto) follow one another in the order of the chakras. I view this coincidence as another indication of the astrological wisdom hidden in the progression of the zodiac, closely resonating with the rising of the serpent fire of kundalini and the generally upward and expansive nature of this opening side of the ATA, the left side of the human body.

VACCA/TAURUS

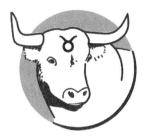

Ruling Planet: Venus (and dwarf planet Eris)
Associated dwarf planet: Ceres
Element: Earth
Quality: Fixed
Numbers: Natural zodiac 2, Hermetic 4
Relative age: Adult (mother)
Gender: Feminine
Zodiac image: Cow or bull
Body part: Throat
Direction: Northeast
Colors: Brown, green
Alchemical metal: Copper
Holidays: May Day, Beltane, Wesak, Cinco de Mayo, Mother's Day
Mythology: Gaia, Venus/Aphrodite, Ceres/Demeter, Eris, Eros and
Psyche, Minos, Pasiphaë, and the Minotaur
Chakra: Fourth, Anahata (unstruck sound), the central heart
Symbol: Green twelve-petaled lotus with a green six-pointed
star
Mantra: *Yang*
Element: Air
Concerns: Love, honor, respect, beauty, harmony
Planets: Venus and Eris

Taurean Astrology

Taurus, the common and familiar name for this fixed earth sign, is usually referred to as the sign of the bull. However, this feminine earth

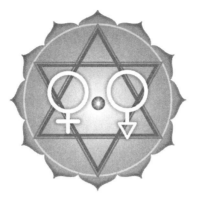

Fig. 2.11. Fourth, or heart, chakra, Anahata

sign, with its strong association with the Great Earth Mother Gaia, is better represented by the cow, whose horns form a crescent, suggesting the crescent Moon, a powerful symbol of the feminine. For this reason, I have added the name Vacca, a Latin word meaning "cow." Vacca/Taurus contains all three stages of woman: maiden, mother, and crone. It is a sign of fertility, sensuality, and the richness of Earth. There can be a deep appreciation of plants, animals, and nature in general. The Moon is exalted in the sign of Vacca/Taurus.

Lovely and loving Venus is the ruling planet of Vacca/Taurus, which connects this sign to the fourth and central heart chakra. Although Venus's other home sign, airy Libra, has a special resonance with the airy nature of the fourth chakra, Venus's earthy love nature is accentuated in this sign. Vacca/Taurus is a fixed earth sign, and its stability and conservative qualities are well known. Like the solid Earth, Vacca has plenty of endurance and perseverance to carry out her tasks and projects to a practical completion.

Taurean Mythology

With Vacca/Taurus and its ruling planet, Venus, we come to a powerfully feminine sign. In regard to feminine signs, it is important to look closely at the dominator values that swept into later Greek myth. Aphrodite and later her Roman counterpart, Venus, suffered the same fate as many of the goddesses, who were demoted in power and married

off to patriarchal gods, who represented the leaders of the new dominator hordes.

Venus

Venus is the goddess of love and, being the ruler of the signs Vacca/
Taurus and Libra, puts the accent on magnetism, sensuality, materialism, and harmony in relationships. Venus represents the qualities a
person might find particularly attractive in others and is symbolic of
how and whom we love. Venus/Aphrodite has a rich, dramatic mythology, especially in the stories of her relationship with her husband,
Hephaestus, and her many lovers, such as Mars/Ares and Mercury/
Hermes. Venus's alchemical metal is lovely copper.

Venus has two sides related to the two signs Libra and Vacca/
Taurus. The Libra side is more attuned to marriage, partnership, and
art, while the Vacca/Taurus side leans more toward sensuality, love
of nature, materialism, and eroticism. Her relationship with passionate Mars is an example of her more Vacca/Taurus side, although their
child, Harmonia, seems to represent a balance of yin and yang. Venus/
Aphrodite is involved in the story of Eris, presented below, and demonstrates how she can seemingly get herself and others in trouble because
of her great beauty and powers of attraction. In Vedic astrology, Venus
is said to be the guru (teacher) of the *asuras,* or demons, which may
refer to her tendency to cause problems associated with excessive desire.
Venus/Aphrodite, like many other goddesses, underwent revisioning at
the hands of the patriarchal Olympians; she was demoted from a goddess of fertility and freedom to an unfaithful wife.

Venus's birth story is rather bizarre. She was born from the foam
that came about when Uranus's severed phallus was thrown into the sea.
Her birth from the sea foam sounds like a sexual metaphor for semen
(sea-men). Her association with the seashell and bivalve is another likely
sexual metaphor.

A significant myth tells of a jealous Venus/Aphrodite, mother of
handsome Eros, who sent her mischievous son to punish the beautiful
mortal Psyche. However, Eros himself fell in love with Psyche. The lov-

ers Eros and Psyche were separated, and Venus/Aphrodite gave Psyche difficult tasks to win back Eros, which she eventually completed and was granted immortality by Jupiter/Zeus. The theme of love and all its attendant complexities is once again dramatized.

Ceres

Ceres, the source for the word *cereal,* is the Roman great nurturing mother like the Greek Demeter. Ceres was the name given to the first and largest asteroid discovered in the asteroid belt between the orbits of Mars and Jupiter. Ceres was reclassified as a dwarf planet in 2006. She has a mythological connection to agriculture, nurturing, food, gardening, and, by extension, to ecology.

The mythology of Ceres/Demeter as mother of the maiden Persephone is activated in this earthy sign of Vacca/Taurus. Via Persephone, Ceres is connected to Pluto/Hades, king of the underworld. The story goes that the naive maiden Persephone was stolen by Hades from Demeter's surface world and taken to be his wife in the underworld. Persephone was given pomegranate seeds to eat by Hades and therefore, for some mysterious reason, probably related to fertility, had to remain there as his wife. Demeter demanded that her daughter be returned to the surface world, and because of her great power over the plant world, Demeter's demands had to be honored. A deal was brokered in which it was decided that Persephone would spend time in each realm, thereby creating summer and winter. This is a profound story with rich symbolic meaning and was the basis of the Greek mysteries of Eleusis, which were enduring rituals of initiation into the secrets of life and death, portrayed in the relationship of mother, daughter, husband, and wife.

Ceres's Special Relationship to Vacca/Taurus

The dwarf planet Ceres and the asteroid belt have an important part to play in the fifth orbit of the solar system, similar to how the musical fifth has a special harmonious part to play in music. In this solar system order that includes Earth, Ceres holds the central position, like the role of Vacca/Taurus in relation to the central heart chakra. In the fact-packed little book by John Martineau, *A Little Book of Coincidence,* he compares Ceres and the asteroid belt to a mirror between the inner four planets and the outer four planets.

Crete and the Bull from the Sea

Another myth that can shed light on the sign of the bull and cow involves the king and queen of Crete. King Minos was born on the island of Crete, the son of Zeus who, in the form of a bull, impregnated the maiden Europa. Minos's wife, Queen Pasiphaë, shared the rulership of their rich and artistic island. Late Greek myth tells that one day a beautiful white bull came ashore out of the waves and Queen Pasiphaë fell in love with it. She had her architect and inventor, Daedalus, create a lifelike cow for her to occupy and was thereby able to conceive a child with the beautiful bull. This child grew to be the half man and half bull named Minotaur, a monster who was kept in a vast, intricate labyrinth, another invention of Daedalus. One way the myth is interpreted portrays the materialistic (from *mater,* meaning "mother") and possessive side of Vacca/Taurus. The beautiful bull from the sea was clearly a divine emanation and was therefore meant to be worshipped in a spiritual fashion, rather than as a possession. The resulting monster was the outcome of a literal materialistic obsession. This tendency toward possessiveness can be seen as a shadow side of the Great Mother archetype.

However, realistically speaking, we can more accurately imagine that the queen of this very gender-balanced culture of ancient Crete, rather than being overly materialistic in the negative sense, was a matron of the arts and had a great deal to do with the beauty and elevated social values associated with this awe-inspiring ancient culture. The monstrous Minotaur was much more likely a creation of the Greeks, who did not appreciate the political power of Minoan Crete. The beautiful and amazing labyrinth, rather than a prison, was an architectural wonder. However, there is a moral to the story: I am reminded, by the myths related to Daedalus's ambivalent inventions, of the story of Dr. Frankenstein's monster, which turned out to be not such a good idea. Indeed, Daedalus's invention of the wings that he and his son, Icarus, used to fly away from Crete led to the death of his son, who flew too close to the Sun, melting the wax on his wings and casting him into the sea.

Eris as Possible Co-ruler of Vacca/Taurus

Eris, similar in many ways to Pluto, is also called a dwarf planet by the astronomical establishment. It is about the same size as Pluto and is located beyond Pluto's orbit. At times, Eris comes just within the orbit of Pluto; at other times, it is quite distant due to its highly elliptical orbit. Eris has a cycle of about 557 years and has been in the sign of Aries during the lives of most of us living today. In 1927, Eris entered the sign of Aries and is presently at about 23 degrees of Aries. It will be in the sign of Aries until 2044, when it enters the sign of Vacca/Taurus. We had a special opportunity at the beginning of the twenty-first century to learn more about Eris since she had been in conjunction with Uranus at around 23 to 24 degrees of Aries for several years. That was a time of rather radically shifting paradigms, wouldn't you say?

The name Eris translates from the Greek as "chaos" or "strife"; her Roman equivalent is Discordia or Discord. Eris appears to have two primary qualities. Like her brother Mars/Ares, she is a fierce warrior who seems to enjoy causing strife and warfare. But the other quality of Eris is that she simply likes motivating folks, sometimes called healthy competition. Although Eris can be associated with either Aries and/or Vacca/Taurus, the primary story associated with Eris is the Judgment of Paris, which involves Aphrodite's prominence in the judgment. This association with Aphrodite/Venus is the basis for my placing Eris in Vacca/Taurus's realm and therefore in the central heart chakra of the ATA.

The Judgment of Paris

In one way of telling this myth, Eris was not invited to a wedding of the divinities, so, in disgust, she threw a golden apple of immortality addressed to "the most beautiful one" into the assembly. Three of the goddesses present claimed the apple, and Zeus commanded Paris, prince of Troy, to be the judge of which of the three goddesses should receive

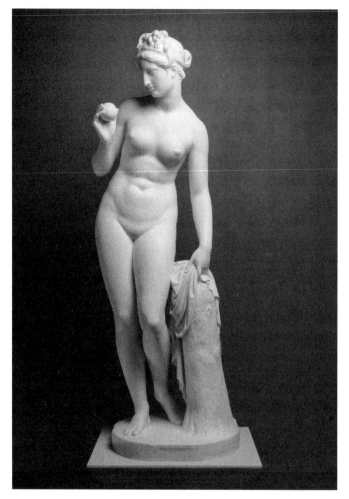

Fig. 2.12. Venus, after winning the beauty contest,
holds the golden apple.
Venus with the Apple by Bertel Thorvaldsen, 1816.

it. Each goddess offered Paris a gift if he were to choose her: Athena offered wisdom (perhaps related to Virgo?), Hera offered power and status (Capricorn?), and Aphrodite offered to give Paris the most beautiful woman in the world (Vacca/Taurus?). Of course, Paris gave the apple to Aphrodite, goddess of love (the apple is associated both with Aphrodite and Hera), and his reward was radiant Helen, indeed said to be the most beautiful woman in the world. There was just one slight problem: Helen was the wife of the Greek king Menelaus of Sparta. The Trojan war was the result.

Thus, it is reasonable to connect the dwarf planet Eris with the sign Vacca/Taurus via the related negative materialistic tendencies of envy, pride, possessiveness, disappointment, and revenge. The golden apple of immortality, like Aphrodite, is irresistible. I wonder, if Paris had chosen Athena's gift of wisdom, could he have placated the other two goddesses and still found his heart's desires without war and his eventual death on the battlefield?

There is an important feminist version of the story of Eris. Brilliant mythologist Jane Ellen Harrison points out that all three goddesses—Aphrodite, Athena, and Hera—were at times portrayed in Greek art as maidens, oftentimes shown carrying fruit and accompanied by Hermes. It was this powerful triple grouping, reminiscent of many portrayals of ancient Greek goddesses, that the later Greek patriarchal society could not abide, so their telling of the story reduced the goddesses to the humiliating situation of competing with one another in a beauty contest. It is likely that Eris is better represented as a goddess of righteous indignation because the women were being reduced from powerful inspiring goddesses to the status of sexual objects and playthings.

I like to think of Eris as an activist for justice, throwing the sought-after apple onto the stage as a brilliant way to disturb the beauty pageant. I am imagining Eris as representing righteous indignation for beings who have been insulted, marginalized, or much worse. A primary theme of the story of Eris and the golden apple is about exclusion and the quest for justice. Henry Seltzer's research on Eris in his book, *The Tenth Planet,* supports this view. According to Seltzer, Eris is often found accented in the astrological charts of people who felt that they were "not invited to the party" and wanted to do something about it.

Eris and the Apple of Immortality

One version of the story says that this magical tree with the golden apples was given to Hera by Gaia as a wedding gift when Hera agreed to marry Zeus. This is perhaps another reason why Hera was not happy to have Paris give Eris's golden apple to Aphrodite. Paris might have done better studying the rich history of the apple, which contains many stories that deserve deep contemplation. It is also notable that the apple is the fruit most resembling the tube torus, a prime geometrical life-form.

When the great triple goddesses are involved, as they must be in the sign of Vacca/Taurus, it is wise to remember that the snake is their totem animal, and fruit, perhaps especially the apple, is symbolic of their juicy fertility. This view of the story should take us back to the time when the goddesses were greatly honored. Later versions of the story denigrate the feminine. The name Taurus the bull, rather than Vacca the cow, for the sign of the Great Earth Mother could be seen in this same light.

Eris, a Modern Story

In the tradition of the wonderful little book *Lost Goddesses of Early Greece* by Charlene Spretnak, I would like to tell a modern version of Eris and the wedding party.

Eris didn't really want to go to that stupid wedding party anyway. Everyone there would be enthralled by the many Hollywood stars and wealthy politicians in attendance, but what really irked her was the way the women would be forced to compete with one another by participating in this degrading ceremony of glamor and opulence.

Then an idea came to Eris. She would make a huge, beautiful package shaped like a golden apple, put it with the wedding gifts, and write on it: "To the most beautiful and powerful woman at the party." Of course, this beautifully wrapped gift caused quite a stir when it came to light. Immediately, everyone started looking around the party at the many very beautiful and elegantly dressed women.

An alpha male stepped forward and reminded everyone that the note also said powerful, and his wife was not only beautiful, but she was also a senator and a likely candidate for vice president. Another man spoke up to say that his date was not only beautiful but also had just won the competition on the *National Idol Singing Contest*.

Soon an argument broke out, and it was suggested that the handsome best man of the wedding should make the choice of who should get the glittering gold gift. It was even suggested that he might have his choice of a date with any single woman at the party when the gift was awarded.

The best man listened to the qualifications and not-so-subtle offers of rewards from the three main candidates, but in his heart he knew that he had been very attracted to the beautiful movie star all along, and after pretending to deliberate a few minutes, he chose the star and handed her the elegantly wrapped package, which she immediately unwrapped to find a cut of raw beef steak.

As the story goes, the best man and the beautiful movie star did go out together, amid vigorous coverage by the tabloids. Later, it was discovered that the movie star was married, and the best man died under suspicious circumstances.

Pandora

There is another tragic example of myth-bending associated with the sign of the Great Mother's sacred cow, Vacca/Taurus. This has to do with the treatment of the creative earth goddess Pandora. Her name Pandora, which means "all gifts," originally referred to Earth Mother Gaia and all the wondrous gifts of Earth, symbolized by her *pithos,* or jar, filled with food and other earthy gifts, like a cornucopia. Instead, the patriarchal myth says that Hephaestus built Pandora, the first woman, like constructing a robot. Her sensuously curved jar was replaced with an angular box filled with sickness, death, and other cruel tricks, which was supposedly released on humankind as a punishment for Prometheus's theft of fire from the gods, which he gave to humans. That female sex robots are now being developed and sold indicates that this misogynist myth is still being enacted. Once again, technology is shown as highly problematic. Aren't technology boxes (computers and smart phones) unleashing trickery and even promoting disease through misinformation? Which has the world on the brink of self-destruction, Pandora's graceful jar or technology's box?

GEMINI

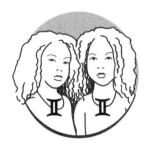

Ruling planet: Mercury
Element: Air
Quality: Mutable
Numbers: Natural zodiac 3, Hermetic 5
Relative age: Youth
Gender: Masculine (or neutral)
Zodiac image: Twins (or lovers)
Body parts: Hands, arms, shoulders, lungs
Direction: Northeast
Colors: Gray, silver, light blue, rainbow colors
Alchemical metal: Mercury (quicksilver)
Holidays: Memorial Day, Father's Day, Pentecost
Mythology: Mercury/Hermes, Dioscuri, Iris, Maia
Chakra: Fifth, Vishuddha (purity), throat
    Symbol: Blue or smoky purple sixteen-petaled lotus with a
       white or blue circle
    Mantra: *Hang*
    Element: Ether
    Concerns: Pure speech, expression, creativity, and
       discrimination
    Planet: Mercury

Geminian Astrology

Gemini is ruled by Mercury/Hermes, who is multitalented and known for
having many names, such as trickster, coyote, messenger, and soul guide.

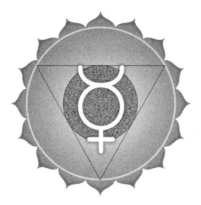

Fig. 2.13. Fifth, or throat, chakra, Vishuddha

Gemini is a talented general communicator, suggesting that this sign can explore multiple subjects. Gemini seems to know at least something interesting about almost everything, allowing folks with this sign prominent to be smart, witty communicators and entertainers. The challenge for Gemini is to find a subject to explore in depth rather than remaining on the surface. Gemini is usually good with wordplay and images. Due to the Hermetic trait of playing with images, Gemini can appear in many guises, like a chameleon. Gemini is also connected to magic.

Twins are the image of Gemini. In Greek myth, the twin half brothers Castor and Polydeukes (or Pollux, the Roman name) were known as the Dioscuri; they were inseparable friends and were symbolic of dualistic thought. In ancient times, this third sign was called the Lovers, revealing the close relationship between love and communication (note the word *intercourse*).

Gemini is the third sign of the natural zodiac, akin to the third person in a group or the child added to the parents, a triangle that brings movement and change. Like the ruler of this sign, Mercury, air sign Gemini is the point of the arrowhead, the mind in flight.

There is another profound message in the imagery of the twins: a great number of primal creation myths from around the world begin with a story of twins. As we will see in chapters 3 and 9, the twin intertwined serpents on Hermes's staff, like the twin tantric channels ida and pingala and the twin strands of the DNA double helix, point toward the inde-scribable impossibility of the beginning of duality from unity and the equally paradoxical creation of unity from duality. This is certainly part of the meaning of Hermes's magical staff: it is used for healing, for making whole. Mercury/Hermes, minister to the divine marriage of the Sun and Moon, is called to the healing task of making the alchemical elixir, the amalgam of silver and gold, also known as the creative union of Cancer and Leo. Hermes is also the midwife to the resulting magical child, which becomes the philosopher's stone, or Herm—Hermes's milestone.

Geminian Mythology
Mercury/Hermes

Mercury, messenger of the gods, is associated with both the clear and the restless mind. Mercury/Hermes has a rich and complex story. Mercury/Hermes's mother, Maia, is the goddess of the mountain cave. Maia (the namesake of our month of May) has a rich mythology, as well, and is one of the stars in the Seven Sisters, or Pleiades. Mercury/Hermes is the messenger to the gods in Olympus; to Pluto/Hades and his queen, Persephone, in the underworld; and to Neptune's and Salacia's emotional watery realm. He is often pictured as the fourth partner of the triple god-desses (such as maiden, mother, and crone; the three graces; the three muses, etc.), and he travels among all these realms. Mercury's alchemical metal is mercury, or quicksilver, the mutable metal.

Mercury is the ruler of two signs, Gemini and Virgo. With the sign Gemini involved, it is Mercury's communication skills and trick-ster nature that are most accented. Mercury, like the busy mind, can be helpful for gathering information and experience but will benefit from focus, depth, and discipline. Mercury is also the ruler of Virgo, which brings out more of his precision and practicality.

Mercury carries the soul over all thresholds and is therefore the hierophant or initiator into new spiritual dimensions. When he is moving in a backward or retrograde manner, Mercury's qualities are especially accented since we then are often bothered by interruptions in the communication process. Mercury/Hermes is known as a guide

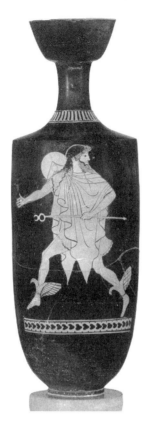

Fig. 2.14. Greek Hermes.
Terracotta oil flask,
circa 475 BCE.

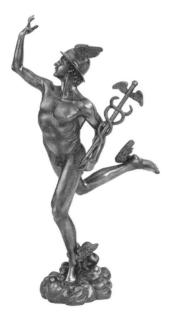

Fig. 2.15. Roman Mercury.
Mercurius by Giovanni da
Bologna, 1580.

to the many realms that attract his wide interest, but his journeys carrying the soul to the underworld after death, into Hades's realm, are especially important.

Mercury, as related to the number 3, is also the third person or minister who presides over the alchemical marriage, so his presence in a sign or house adds to that sign's or house's ability to merge the various parts of the psyche into an integrated whole.

The following are some of the most well-known of Mercury/Hermes's roles, with brief descriptions:

Messenger. As speaker and carrier of messages, he has a neutral role. He carries messages for all the other divinities without bias. He carries the staff or talking stick of democracy. Mercury/Hermes is associated with the fifth, or throat, chakra in the tantric system. His caduceus/staff can be viewed as representing the chakra system and is an especially favored symbol in the ATA system.

Guide. Hermes carries the soul or psyche into many realms but is especially known as the psychopomp, or guide of the soul, into Hades's underworld.

Midwife. His mother's name is Maia, which means "midwife." One of Hermes's epithets is Hermes Maia, and he is shown as male midwife, for instance, in the birth of Dionysus from Zeus's thigh. Socrates refered to his philosophy as based on the maieutic method, which suggests asking questions in dialogue to birth the truth rather than to teach as an expert. This is certainly a philosophy guided by Hermes.

Trickster/fool. Like Coyote in Native American Indian lore, Hermes plays tricks on everyone, mortals and divinities alike.

Seducer. Hermes has his own brand of sexuality, perhaps indicated by his many unusual and bizarre children, such as Hermaphroditus, Pan, and Priapus. See the strange and wonderful book *Hermes and His Children* by Rafael Lopez-Pedraza for more information on this part of Hermes's story.

Hierophant. As the alchemical agent and minister of the divine marriage, Hermes is the third party, the synthesizer or connector. He is portrayed as the third party in the alchemical marriage of the silver Moon and golden Sun.

Secret keeper. As in hermetically sealed, Hermes is the namesake of hidden or occult knowledge. The Hermetic tradition is based on the Egyptian Thoth; in this tradition, Hermes is called Hermes Trismegistus, the thrice great or thrice born. Also see Martin Heidegger's hermeneutical phenomenology for another view of Hermes's role in philosophy. The word, *secretary* literally means "keeper of secrets." Hermes is the divine secretary.

Companion to the triple goddesses. Hermes is cast in the role of completing the feminine trinity of goddesses to create the quaternity.

Thief. See Norman O. Brown's book *Hermes the Thief* for a scholarly treatment of Hermes related to his role as trickster and thief. Hermes, for example, as a child stole cattle from his half brother Apollo and hid them.

Trader at the boundaries. Hermes is the divinity of merchants, especially those who trade among groups and countries. He is cunning and a good businessman. He is the primal translator/ interpreter. Also a good salesman and ad man, Hermes is the original spin doctor.

Hermes and the herm. The rock or pile of rocks used to indicate the way on a road was considered a divinity of the road and travel. This rock became the milestone and eventually the phallic stone, or herm. Thus, with Mercury's influence, Gemini is a sign related to movement and being on the road exploring.

Dioscuri, the Twins

Although Dioscuri means "sons of Zeus," the two sons, Castor and Pollux/Polydeukes, although inseparable, were actually half brothers with the same mother but different fathers. Polydeukes was an immortal son of Zeus and brother of Helen of Troy. Zeus mated with Polydeukes's mother, Leda, in the form of a swan. The almost twins participated in many battles and adventures together, eventually being placed in the sky by Zeus as the constellation Gemini. Polydeukes was immortal, and Castor was mortal; because they were so close, they worked out a deal whereby they could share their abilities and spend equal time on Earth and among the divinities. Clearly, the metaphor of unity and duality is well portrayed by the Dioscuri.

Maia

Hermes's mother, Maia, adds a rich imaginal realm to the mythic background of the sign Gemini. Maia and her six sisters are located near the constellation of Gemini, in the star cluster known as the Seven Sisters, or the Pleiades. Maia, the oldest daughter, was said to be the wisest and kindest of these daughters of Atlas, holder of the heavens. Zeus and Maia gave birth to their precocious son, Hermes, in a cave on Mt. Cyllene in Arcadia. As mentioned above, the Greek word *maia* means "midwife," and the images of birth and birthing are symbolized by Maia's dark cave. The similar-sounding and related, if not identical, name Maya evokes the Great Goddess of the swirling phenomenal world of Hinduism and also the mother of the Buddha. The parallels between Hermes and Buddha are intriguing, as is the connection to the Central American Mayan culture.

Mother Maia lends her name to our month of May, with its springtime images of fertility and the maypole dance. Gemini, related to the number 3, can be imagined as the Taurus couple joined by their minister/son, Mercury/Hermes, the central post or World Tree around which the dancing maypole couples interweave their karmic ribbons, like the dance of the phenomenal world, tied to the central unmanifest *bindu,* or dot. Imagine Zeus embracing starry Maia in their night sky cave as the Vacca/Taurus couple, with baby Hermes making three.

CANCER

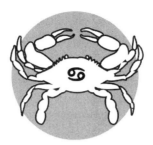

Ruling planet: Moon
Associated dwarf planet: Ceres
Associated asteroid: Juno
Element: Water
Quality: Cardinal
Numbers: Natural zodiac 4, Hermetic 6
Relative age: Adult
Gender: Feminine
Zodiac image: Crab
Body parts: Stomach, breasts, uterus
Direction: North
Colors: Silver, white, pale blue, pearl
Alchemical metal: Silver
Holidays: Independence Day, Summer Solstice
Mythology: Selene, Endymion, Mary, Oceanus, Diana/Artemis, Venus/Aphrodite, Soma
Chakra: Sixth, Ajna (command), brow or third eye
  Symbol: Blue-violet two-petaled lotus
  Mantra: *Aum* or *thang*
  Element: Sound
  Concerns: Insight, intuition, compassion
  Planet: Moon

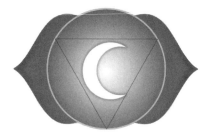

Fig. 2.16. Sixth, or brow, chakra, Ajna

Cancerian Astrology

Cancer, the cardinal water sign, is related to the goddess of the sea. Cancer is a very nurturing and feminine water sign. Traditionally connected to the home and comfort, Cancer thrives on feeling secure. While all three water signs like merging and forming deep emotional bonds, Cancers can have a hard shell, like a crab, as protection due to their great sensitivity and vulnerability.

The Moon is the ruler of the sign of Cancer, and Lady Luna strongly colors this sign of the crab. The Moon is the symbol of the silver queen in alchemy, while the Sun is the golden king. Thus, Sun in Cancer has an inherent quality of alchemical union, bringing together the king and the queen, gold and silver. This psychic marriage offers the potential for profound integration and gives all the folks born with the Sun in this sign inherent gender balance.

Since it is ruled by the Moon, with its three phases of new, full, and old, Cancer is associated with all the triple goddesses: maidens, mothers, and crones. Selene is the goddess of the Moon for the Greeks. Cancer's relationship with the stomach and breasts places an accent on food and nurturing. Thus, the asteroid Juno and dwarf planet Ceres have resonance with Cancer because they are also nurturing mother goddesses, with the feeding and nursing of children accented. Artemis, a maiden goddess, is often portrayed with a crescent Moon, as is Mother Mary. Artemis is known for her care of children and is also related to many divinities of the ocean and other bodies of water. Oceanus and Tethys, Titan divinities of the waters, had numerous offspring, and Artemis had many of their daughters as her followers. Aphrodite, goddess of love, is portrayed as born from the sea, and Venus is comfortable in the sign of Cancer.

As the cardinal, or prime, water sign, Cancer is the great mother of the ocean, which is resonant with the embryonic waters of the uterus, as is all life born in the fertile sea. Oceanus and Tethys were, for the Greeks, a primal couple, and their many children represent the ocean, teeming with life.

Casting reflected light on the sign Cancer, Selene, goddess of the Moon, and her lover, Endymion, the setting Sun, also had many children, like the fertile ocean. Their fifty daughters are named the Menai and appear to correspond with the fifty months (or moons) of the Olympiad, a time period related to the Olympic games (Endymion was also the king of Olympia). The Moon and the Sun are both historically connected to the keeping of time.

Cancer carries connotations of this flowing element, including waters of the womb and lunar white milk from the breasts. Indeed, our Milky Way Galaxy was imagined by the ancient Greeks and Romans as milk spraying from the breasts of the goddess Juno/Hera. Galaxy comes from the Greek word *gala,* which means "milk." The glyph for the sign Cancer is shaped like the number 69 and has been compared to the spiral shape of our Milky Way Galaxy. Cancer is the cardinal sign of nourishment, ruling the breasts as dispensers of milk and the stomach as digestion.

Independence Day is the holiday during this sign of the great water mother. It can be viewed as a celebration of our country's separation from Mother England and hence is rife with mother-child symbolism. Cancer is the fourth sign of the natural zodiac, and the number 4 is related to the square, the home, quaternity, and completion of the trinity. Its multiples of 4, 8, and 12 are the numbers of the sexual water signs, ruling the breasts, genitals, and feet. The Cancer Moon is an oval and like the ovum welcomes the milky white semen (or sea-men?), and there is a deep aura of oceanic fertility in both Lady Luna and the sign of the crab.

Cancerian Mythology
Soma, God of the Moon
According to Hindu myth, Soma, god of the Moon, is the son of Varuna, lord of the oceans. In this story, during each lunar cycle the

Moon is filled from the oceans by Surya, the Sun. As the Moon waxes, she fills with nectar, and as the Moon wanes, the nectar becomes food for the immortals. Daksha was father of the twenty-seven or twenty-eight goddesses of the *nakshatras,* the lunar mansions of Vedic astrology, which were given by Daksha to Soma as a gift. Soma, the Moon god, visits one of the goddesses each night, and it is said that beautiful Rohini, the fourth nakshatra, which is ruled by the Moon and Venus, was Soma's favorite. This, of course, made for jealousy among the other twenty-six goddesses. Soma was a bit of a rascal and also got himself in trouble by eloping with Tara, the wife of Jupiter. When it was discovered that she was pregnant with Soma's child, this caused a great divine uproar. The baby was named Budha or Mercury and, fortunately, was so cute and charming that Jupiter accepted him as his child, and Soma was forgiven. This is a story perhaps suggesting that Mercury or small mind is the rather naughty offspring of Soma or big mind.

Selene and Endymion

Selene, the Greek Moon goddess, fell in love with Endymion, who was, according to various stories, either a handsome shepherd, a king of Olympia, or an astronomer/astrologer; in any case, he was a person who adored the Moon nightly. Selene found Endymion so beautiful that she asked his father, Zeus, to make him stay forever youthful so she could love him in this perfect form. So, Zeus put Endymion into perpetual sleep so that Selene could visit him every evening in his suspended state. Somehow, Selene and Endymion still managed to have fifty daughters, which, as mentioned above, seems to relate to the time period of fifty months called the Olympiad. The story of Selene and her sleeping lover has touched the imagination of many ancient and modern poets and artists.

Artemis

Artemis is primarily known as a virgin goddess living in the wilderness and is often shown accompanying the new crescent Moon, but Artemis also has a mother form that portrays her with a multitude of breasts. She is at times a midwife, as she was for her brother, Apollo, and at other times she is a caretaker of animals and adolescent girls. Later myth identified Diana, the Roman Moon Goddess, as the equivalent of Artemis and the lover of Endymion. Artemis is definitely a goddess who is associated with women and the Moon, especially the wilder aspects of femininity. This is not necessarily the stereotype of the nurturing, home-loving Cancer person, but rather, this myth represents another side of Cancer. There is also a sleepy, unconscious quality carried by the Moon and Cancer represented by the union of Selene and Endymion.

Mother Mary

In relationship with the Great Mother archetype, Cancer has a certain affinity with Mary, mother of Jesus. The name Mary reveals a link with the sea, and Mother Mary is often portrayed with the crescent Moon and called the Star of the Sea. Being the mother of Jesus, she can be seen as the womb of all life, the great ocean of compassion, and is associated with the sixth, or brow, chakra, symbolic of higher consciousness. This fourth sign, Cancer, is the original home as womb and birthplace of the nectar of everlasting life, Christ consciousness, and enlightenment. The Holy Grail can be understood as Mary's crescent womb, chalice of the life-blood of Jesus.

Venus/Aphrodite

Venus/Aphrodite is said to have been born from the sea foam arising from the severed genitals of Uranus. The stories vary, placing this occurrence offshore on one of two Greek islands, either Cythera or Cyprus. Regardless, this reflects her association with the sea. Aphrodite's connection to water and fertile female sexuality is resonant with the Moon and Cancer's feminine qualities.

Oceanus and Tethys

Oceanus (oceans) and Tethys (fresh waters) were Titans, born from Gaia (Earth) and Uranus (the heavens), and represented the oceans and fresh waters. Uranus, namesake of the heavens and father of the oceans, demonstrates that the ancients identified these two realms: heavens and oceans. The children of Oceanus and Tethys include a multitude of sea beings and all the beings of rivers and streams of water. Their flowing waters teeming with life contribute to Cancer's rich, wide, oceanic qualities.

LEO

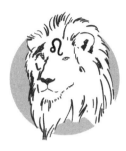

Ruling planet: Sun
Associated asteroids: Pallas, Vesta
Element: Fire
Quality: Fixed
Numbers: Natural zodiac 5, Hermetic 7
Relative age: Adult
Gender: Masculine
Zodiac image: Lion or lioness
Body parts: Heart, solar plexus, back, spine
Direction: Northwest
Colors: Gold, scarlet
Alchemical metal: Gold
Holiday: Lammas
Mythology: Dionysus, Ariadne, Apollo, Amaterasu, Surya, Vesta, Pallas Athene, Helios
Chakra: Seventh, Sahasrara (thousand petals), crown
   Symbol: Multicolored multipetaled lotus
   Mantra: *Aum* or *om*
   Element: Light
   Concerns: Connecting with the source or the divine, beyond the separate self
   Planet: Sun

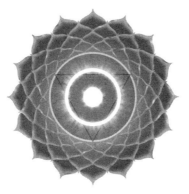

Fig. 2.17. Seventh, or crown, chakra, Sahasrara

Leonine Astrology

Leo is a fixed fire sign and in the zodiac is represented by the lion, known as the king of the beasts. In the case of a woman, the lioness is perhaps more appropriate. The lioness, although also powerful, is the provider and caretaker of her pride. Leo is known for being playful and liking children. Leo is the fifth sign of the natural order of the zodiac, which is of the quintessence. Whereas the Moon is related to silver, Leo is the sign of the golden king or queen and is ruled by the Sun, the "star" of our solar system. Leo is the actor of the zodiac and likes drama and being on stage, especially as the star and center of attention. Leo is known for being generous and, like the Sun, shares his or her radiance with everyone.

Although there is a connection in the sign Leo to the mythology of the solar divinities, including Helios and Apollo, I find the mythology of Dionysus and his dramatic ecstatic path even more fitting. On the cusp of the sign of the lion, with its solar fire, and at the end of the lunar water of the sign of the crab, we have the perfect antipode to the cusp between Capricorn and Aquarius. Cancer and Leo form the silver and gold alchemical couple and from their union comes the ecstasy. In yogic terms, from the union of being and consciousness comes *ananda,* or bliss. This is not something to be attained but simply realized: being is conscious and hence naturally blissful. In tantric terms, sexual union and orgasm is a remembrance of the overall state of existence. In other words, the unmanifest and the manifest are one. The black hole and the white hole are two sides of the dimensionless dot called the bindu. This Sankrit word means "point" or "dot," but it can also be translated as "not (*bin*) two (*du*)." This meaning or wordplay was shared with me by my artist friend, sage, and self-avowed rascal, Prasanna.

Lammas

The sign Leo contains the pagan holiday Lammas, celebrated on or around August first, which is a cross-quarter time between the summer solstice and the autumnal equinox. Coming near the midpoint of Leo, although the weather in the Northern Hemisphere is still often quite hot, the Leo cross-quarter time can be subtly recognized as the beginning of autumn. Traditionally, the first harvest of wheat was made into a loaf of bread and shared with the community at this time. In terms of the tantric cycle, the bliss of the dramatic sacred marriage of the Sun and the Moon is like the quintessential summer high, reversed now in Hermetic Leo, into the downward, distributing path: the fruits of the Sun and Moon tree are now ripe and ready to be harvested. The offspring of the alchemical union of masculine and feminine is a wonderful energy that can now be distributed to the rest of the subtle body. The fullness of summer is part of Leo's royal presence and from it radiates forth Leo's generosity.

Leonine Mythology

As mentioned above, radiant Apollo is often identified with the Sun; however, his intellectual light can be blinding, so I tend to associate him more with the sign opposite to Leo, scientific Aquarius. Leo is more at home with Dionysus's story. In Greek myth, Dionysus is the divinity of the dramatic stage, vine, and the wine. Along with the wine comes the ecstatic trance state that is a central part of Dionysus's story. Born of Zeus and Demeter, Dionysus, like the vine, goes through profound transformation as the grape becomes the wine. In a story that is noticeably similar to that of the Egyptian solar king Osiris and his wife and sister, Isis, Dionysus is killed by the Titans and torn into pieces.

His parts were gathered together by either Demeter or Apollo. Zeus took the heart of Dionysus and gave it to Semele, a goddess of Earth and the Moon, who became pregnant with the renewed Dionysus. Once again, embryonic Dionysus is almost destroyed when Semele is incinerated by Zeus but is saved from the flames by Zeus and sewn into his thigh. Hermes as midwife received baby Dionysus as he was reborn from the thigh of his father, Zeus. When mature, one of Dionysus's quests was to visit the underworld, where he brought back to the surface world his mother, Semele. Dionysus's very dramatic and eventful life included living in the wilderness with the wild female maenads and the sensual male satyrs and also presided over festivals of the poets and playwrights. Clearly the gift of his sacred wine was a boon to a wide range of humans, although it is also clear that there was a price to pay, symbolized by Dionysus's association with the underworld.

It is apparent that Dionysus's wine was especially helpful to women. The epitome of Dionysus's care is shown in his marriage to Ariadne, royal princess of Crete. After Ariadne helped the Athenian Theseus find his way out of the labyrinth, using her ball of yarn, they eloped, but Theseus abandoned her on the island of Naxos, which happened to be one of Dionysus's cult centers. On Naxos, Dionysus fell in love with Ariadne, and they married.

Although there are several stories about Ariadne's fate, her association with ecstatic dance stands out. The archetypal architect and inventor Daedalus built her a dance floor in Crete, and when Theseus escaped from the labyrinth, they danced together in a great celebration. Likewise, when Dionysus and Ariadne were married, ecstatic dance was emphasized. To this day, in celebrations of Ariadne, dancing is the primary expression. Ariadne is certainly a fitting female archetype for ecstatic Leo, as dance is a perfect dramatic expression of how to find our way either into the center or out of the labyrinth of life. Wine and dance make a lovely couple, and, notably, the heroic warrior types, like Theseus, are not known for their dancing skills.

As another reference to Leo's royalty and association with the seventh, or crown, chakra, Ariadne is also known for her beautiful crown.

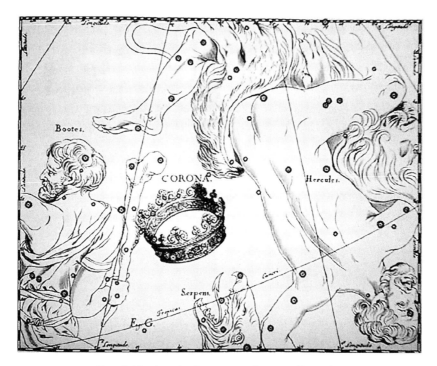

Fig. 2.18. Ariadne's crown, Corona Borealis,
by Johannes Hevelius, from *Prodromus Astronomiae*.

One version of the story says that Theseus, in proving himself to Ariadne's father, King Minos, retrieved from the depths of the sea the golden crown created by Hephaestus and gave it to Ariadne. Another version of the story says that Dionysus gave Ariadne the beautiful crown and, as a tribute to her, placed the crown in the sky as the constellation Corona Borealis.

Turnaround

With the sign Leo the height of attainment of the cycle is reached, either of complete egohood, death of the false notion of a separate self, or, more likely, something in between. The radiant golden king or queen either distributes his or her selfish glory on the wheel of royal succession or becomes the servant of his or her people—either Henry VIII or good King Wenceslas.

After reaching the top of the ascending half of the cycle of the ATA zodiac, the energy and lessons of this apparent journey are distributed back down through the chakras. Following the symbolism represented by the cycle of the ida and pingala channels, the "individual" continues the slow evolution as revolution on the wheel of the dual nadis. Thus, the journey down through the remaining five astrological signs, from Virgo to Capricorn, is telling the story of return and distribution, which completes this cycle.

Like Shiva and Parvati united, the royal marriage of the Sun in Leo and the Moon in Cancer represents the union of the sixth and seventh chakras. Now we start the downward, distributing path at the fifth chakra and the sign of Virgo.

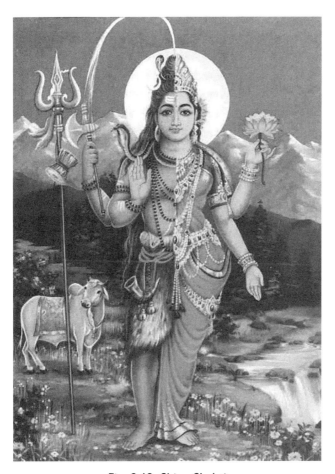

Fig. 2.19. Shiva Shakti

VIRGO

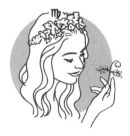

Ruling planet: Mercury
Associated asteroids: Vesta, Pallas, Chiron
Element: Earth
Quality: Mutable
Numbers: Natural zodiac 6, Hermetic 8
Relative age: Youth
Gender: Feminine
Zodiac image: Virgin goddess holding a stalk of grain or corn
Body part: Intestines
Direction: West
Colors: Brown, white, gray, blue
Alchemical metal: Mercury
Holiday: Woman's Equality Day
Mythology: Artemis, Hestia, Vesta, Athena, Hygieia, Iris
Chakra: Fifth, Vishuddha (purity), throat, seed mantra *hang*
    Symbol: Blue or smoky purple sixteen-petaled lotus with a
      white or blue circle
    Element: Ether
    Concerns: Pure speech, expression, creativity, and
      discrimination

Virgoan Astrology

Virgo is the sign of strong and discriminating Goddesses. Excellent mental abilities allow Virgo to be precise and practical, especially about work, health, and service. This allows a Virgo person to be a clear

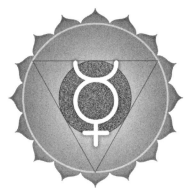

Fig. 2.20. Fifth, or throat, chakra, Vishuddha

communicator with a great deal of attention to detail. Virgo is a mutable earth sign, which may sound rather paradoxical, but another way to say it is that, with Mercury as ruler, Virgo combines mutable mental abilities with precise, practical, down-to-earth abilities. Because a Virgo person can be so discerning, she or he can also be critical of self and others. Virgo combines some rather divergent qualities, including powerful feminine energy that can manifest as healing care, service, and protecting the young.

Virgoan Mythology

Virgo symbolism contains three main and quite different archetypes: Artemis, Hestia, and Athena.

Artemis is the Greek goddess most resonant with the sign of Virgo. In myth she is a powerful goddess of the wilderness and a huntress. She is protective of her privacy. Artemis was especially a guardian and wild leader of preteen girls. There is an impressive story related to Artemis that demonstrates some of her virginal boundary keeping. It is told that the great hunter and Theban hero Actaeon, who was a student of Chiron, was in the wilderness with his hunting dogs when they happened upon Artemis in her bath. Artemis turned Actaeon into a stag and his own dogs devoured him! I have an ancient coin from Ephesus, famous home of Artemis's temple. On one side of the coin there is a kneeling stag and on the other side is a bee. Artemis was associated with bees, and like the bee, she has both sweetness and a sting.

Virgo relates to the Greek goddess Hestia, who rules the home fires and the central hearth of the home, and also the Roman goddess Vesta, a version of the virgin as keeper of the sacred flame in the center of the city of Rome.

A third goddess can also be associated with the sign of Virgo. It is said that Aphrodite, the Greek goddess of love, held sway over all the divinities with the exception of Artemis, Hestia, and Athena. Hence, the protector warrior goddess Athena also has a place in this sign of the virgin. All three of these powerful goddesses lend their strong archetypal presence to the sign of Virgo.

In learning about the planetary beings related to Virgo, it is good to pay special attention to the sixth house and the asteroids Vesta and Pallas, since all these relate strongly to the sign of Virgo. The sixth house, like the sixth sign, Virgo, has to do with work, service, and health.

Pallas Athene, another name for Athena, relates to the archetype of feminine protective power, an energy that goes beyond the usual definition of femininity to include protection of the higher values of the culture.

Beyond the home and hearth, Virgo's resonant sixth house is related to health and thereby additionally associated with the goddess daughter of Asclepias, Hygieia, whose motto is that health is based on day-to-day balanced living rather than on the more heroic ideal of the doctor as fixer.

Iris

Being a feminine messenger, related to the wind and air, Iris is another good archetypal image for the combination of sign Virgo and planet Mercury. A messenger goddess, Iris is winged and fleet of foot. The word *iris* means "rainbow," and Iris is known to use a rainbow to travel between Earth and the abode of the divinities on Mount Olympus. Although Iris carries messages for all the divinities, she is especially associated with Hera and is said to rest each evening by Hera's couch, with her sandals on, ready to go on a mission at a moment's notice. Connected to the winds, Iris is often carried by them on her travels. Like Hermes, one of her duties is to travel to the underworld. Once in Hades's realm, she gathers water from the River Styx in a golden goblet, which is used by the divinities during the swearing of their most solemn oaths. The colorful poetic images related to Iris, such as rainbow, eye, and female messenger, open another dimension of the way Virgo manifests in the world and connects her strongly to the subtlety of the fifth chakra and the ether element. The virginity of this sign is also connected to the Hermetic numerology of the number 8, which places Virgoan mythology beyond the physical into the realm of ethereal spiritual servant.

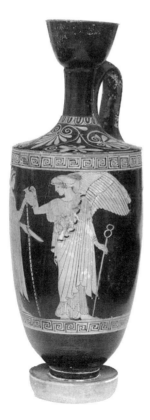

Fig. 2.21. Iris, the winged messenger goddess.

Terracotta oil flask, circa 475 BCE.

LIBRA

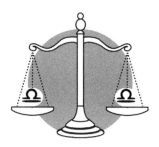

Ruling planet: Venus (Eris)
Associated asteroid: Juno
Element: Air
Quality: Cardinal
Numbers: Natural zodiac 7, Hermetic 9
Relative age: Adult
Gender: Masculine
Zodiac images: Scales, balance
Body parts: Hips, kidneys, lower back
Direction: West
Colors: Green, blue
Alchemical metal: Copper
Holiday: Columbus Day/Indigenous People's Day
Mythology: Venus/Aphrodite, Urania, Athena, Vulcan/Hephaestus,
Juno/Hera, Eris
Chakra: Fourth, Anahata (unstruck sound), the central heart
Symbol: Green twelve-petaled lotus with a green six-pointed
star
Mantra: *Yang*
Element: Air
Concerns: Love, honor, respect, beauty, harmony

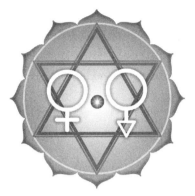

Fig. 2.22. Fourth, or heart, chakra, Anahata

Libran Astrology

The sign Libra begins at the autumnal equinox, at the balance point between summer and winter (in the Northern Hemisphere), and is a prime example of the balancer of opposites. Libras are known for being fair and diplomatic. As a consequence, there can be a tendency to go overboard, wanting to be fair and just in all their dealings. Also, they likely have an inherent sense of artistic placement and know intuitively when things are out of place or not arranged optimally. Libras often have a good musical ear for the same reason, a natural appreciation for harmony and balance. If the Libra person can relax a bit and not try to keep everything in balance, she or he can deeply enjoy beauty and the finer things of life. Since lovely Venus is the ruling planet of Libra, there is a natural flair and grace in relationships, and the Libra person can bring an artistic touch to this realm as well.

Libra is the seventh sign of the natural zodiac and partakes of the good fortune of this lucky number. Seven is a number related to the colors of the rainbow and the seven notes in a musical scale, which are the colors and sounds of Libra's artistic temperament. In the Alchemical Tantric Arrangement, Libra becomes the ninth sign, and this number's quality as the largest single digit speaks of Libra's extra importance because of its relationship to the central heart chakra, centered between the upper three and lower three chakras. The central heart proves the insight that, no matter the question, love is the answer.

The symbol for Libra is the balance and it is the only zodiac sign not represented by an animal. It is symbolic of the scales of justice and has connotations of fairness, balance, harmony, and discrimination. Libra comes at the time of the equinox and is pointing toward this yearly balance between day and night. The shape of the Libra glyph and can be seen as representing the central bulge of our spiral galaxy when seen from the edge. Libra is a cardinal sign, and the four cardinal signs resonate with the Milky Way Galaxy since they are related to the solstices and equinoxes and are therefore connected to the north–south axis of Earth.

Libran Mythology

Besides Venus/Aphrodite, Libra is also associated with the husband of Aphrodite, the smith and artist Hephaestus, who is credited with many inventions and works of art. Libra, as an intellectual air sign, has a strong connection to mental prowess, along with artistic and relationship skills.

Juno

Queen and royal mother, wife, and gifted practitioner of the arts and crafts, as balance to her royal husband, Jupiter, Juno symbolizes graceful power in relationships. Although Juno/Hera was presented in Olympian myth as primarily a jealous wife, an older, deeper level of her story tells of her great skill, power, and presence in a relationship. She and Jupiter/Zeus represent the royal marriage and the importance of their gender balance as co-rulers. The quality of royal partnership is emphasized by Juno/Hera's close association with the Great Mother Goddess and the power and authority thereof. This royal marriage symbolizes the ability to appreciate the hidden parts of the psyche, integrate, and realize wholeness and union within oneself and in a relationship.

Eris

Although it might seem difficult at first to see the connection between Libra and Eris, a goddess often connected with strife, when we focus more on her love of justice we can see her similarity with Venus/Aphrodite in the use of a calculating feminine approach to overcoming opposition. Eris used trickery to prove her point in the Judgment of Paris myth, and Libra's balance can be seen as representing the scales of justice. The recent transit of Uranus over Eris around 2016 and the huge response of women to President Trump and other men who misuse women suggests a powerful example of Eris's involvement. Time will tell which signs astrologers will associate with the planet Eris; however, there is certainly a basis for placing this goddess with a love for justice in the fourth chakra.

SCORPIO

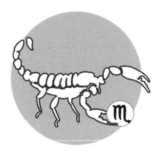

Ruling planet: Pluto (Mars)
Element: Water
Quality: Fixed
Numbers: Natural zodiac 8, Hermetic 10
Relative age: Youth
Gender: Feminine
Zodiac image: Scorpion
Body parts: Genitals, colon, anus
Direction: Southeast
Colors: Orange, rust, red-orange
Alchemical metal: Plutonium (iron)
Holidays: Halloween, All Saints' Day, Day of the Dead, United Nations Day, Election Day, Veteran's/Armistice Day
Mythology: Pluto/Hades, Persephone, Hecate, Mars/Ares, Shiva, Kali, Vesta
Chakra: Third, Manipura (jeweled city), navel, solar plexis
   Symbol: Yellow ten-petaled lotus with a fiery red triangle
   Mantra: *Rang*
   Element: Fire
   Concerns: Power, control, will, strength, focus, force

Scorpionic Astrology

Scorpio has several images that convey its intense and soulful traits. The first is the scorpion with its notorious sting. Folks who have to live around this scorpion energy come to know about the shocking and pain-

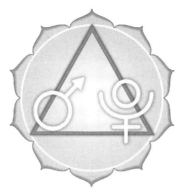

Fig. 2.23. Third, or navel, chakra, Manipura

ful "sting" in the form of verbal and energetic attacks. A common story regarding the scorpion says that it can kill itself with its own stinger. Anyone with the sign of Scorpio prominent in his or her chart has some strong connection to death. Just as the scorpion might be found hiding under a desert rock to escape the heat, likewise Scorpio is known for being secretive. It is easy to wonder what might lie just below the surface of all the well-hidden, powerful emotions of this hot water sign.

Sometimes the spider, and especially the female black widow spider, is associated with Scorpio. The black widow's black color, red-orange hourglass mark on its abdomen, sticky web, and poisonous bite contribute to its frightening Halloween aura, a holiday under Scorpio's purview.

Another image for Scorpio is the snake, especially the desert rattler. Again, we see the dangerous attributes, and in addition, we can see the quality of transformation in the snake's shedding of its skin. There are other connotations to the snake that relate it to the sign of Scorpio. Snakes, which often live in holes in the ground, are traditionally connected to Scorpio's hidden and underworld associations. And, of course, the snake and Cosmic Serpent suggest intense energy, including kundalini and the mysterious serpentine DNA molecule.

The high-flying eagle, with its penetrating eyesight, is also associated with Scorpio, based on this sign's ability to see deeply into any situation or persona. Scorpios make good investigators and detectives. Scorpio can also be described as insightful; however, although they may appear to have lofty ideas, their worldly wisdom is often based on shadowy living experiences.

Finally, Scorpio is associated with the phoenix, a mythical bird that flies high, is destroyed in its funeral pyre, and is reborn from the ashes. This association points to the apocalyptic quality of this eighth sign of the natural zodiac, with connotations of infinity, death and rebirth, the higher octave, and transmutation. They have the ability to "burn their bridges," to move on from an experience and not look back.

Both Mars and Pluto are identified as the ruling planets of Scorpio. Historically, Scorpio was ruled by Mars. When Pluto was discovered, it became the main ruler of Scorpio instead, lending a profound connection with death and the underworld to the meaning of this sign. Scorpio remains resonant with Mars and its connotations of war and outgoing dynamic energy.

Scorpionic Mythology

The Greek myths about Pluto/Hades and Persephone are truly fitting for Scorpio. Of the three Olympian brothers, Pluto/Hades is the ruler of the underworld, while Jupiter/Zeus rules the sky and Neptune/Poseidon rules the seas. Hades abducted the maiden Persephone from the surface world while she was gathering flowers and carried her to his underworld domain. Persephone's mother, Demeter/Ceres, goddess of the surface of Earth, went in search of her daughter and in her anguish caused Earth's vegetation to perish. (Could this myth have relevance to our times of climate change and environmental degradation?) While in the underworld, Persephone ate of the pomegranate, which sealed her fate, requiring her always to return to Hades's realm for part of the year. The seed-filled pomegranate is a rich, fertile image, suggesting the ovary filled with eggs, and the blood-red juice of the fruit is symbolic of living tissue and dying menstrual blood. The suggestion is that sexuality and its attaching tendencies are part of why Persephone needed to return to the underworld.

There are many levels of meaning to this profound story, in keeping with Scorpio's depth and intensity. Scorpio is on the opposite side of the zodiac from earthy Vacca/Taurus, a sign associated with Persephone's mother, Demeter/Ceres. In one sense, Scorpio is a sign of union, combining the high-flying eagle and phoenix with the low-crawling spider and serpent—spirit and soul, to use James Hillman's dichotomy. Scorpio tends toward the darker side of the dualities of life-death, surface-underworld, literal-symbolic.

Hecate is the crone and wise elder aspects of the triple goddess. Some would say she is part of the archetype of the witch. In his etching *The Night of Enitharmon's Joy,* William Blake portrays Hecate with her two other aspects and some associated animals—especially animals of the night, like the owl, bat, and serpent. The sign of Scorpio contains a good deal of Hecate's presence as well as the presence of the maiden Persephone and Queen Persephone. In an older stratum of myth, Hecate was the ruler of three realms: the Moon, the sky, and the underworld. Scorpio's inherent soulful journey runs parallel to Persephone's journey from curious, naive maiden to the depths of hell and back. She reunites with her mother and also becomes the queen of the underworld and eventually identifies with the wise, magical grandmother, Hecate, who was able to observe Persephone's abduction and help bring about the integration of her two roles as daughter and queen/wife. The Scorpio theme of the highest together with the lowest is once again demonstrated by Persephone and the goddess Hecate.

Mars/Ares, god of war, is the older ruler of Scorpio, and some of his brash and direct approach is part of Scorpio's qualities. Shiva and Kali, god and goddess of destruction in the Hindu trinity, can also be related to the sign of Scorpio; there is clearly the spiritual perspective of destroying delusion and the false belief in a separate self in their stories. The combination of highest spirituality with death and destruction places Shiva and Kali in the Scorpio camp.

Scorpio's connection with death and dying is ultimately related to the phrase *die before you die,* as in experience a spiritual death and transformation before your physical death. And it also asks the question: "Death, where is your sting?" The very best use of Scorpio's symbolism is to die to the false notion of a separate self. If you ponder this deeply, it will become clear that the "you" that is not cannot do anything to make itself absent.

SAGITTARIUS

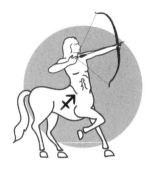

Ruling planet: Jupiter
Associated asteroids: Juno, Chiron
Element: Fire
Quality: Mutable
Numbers: Natural zodiac 9, Hermetic 11
Relative age: Elder
Gender: Masculine
Zodiac image: Centaur archer
Body part: Thighs
Direction: South
Colors: Purple, dark blue, red
Alchemical metal: Tin
Holiday: Thanksgiving Day
Mythology: Jupiter/Zeus, Juno/Hera, Chiron
Chakra: Second, Svadisthana (one's own abode), sacral center, genitals

Symbol: Orange six-petaled lotus

Mantra: *Vang*

Element: Water, represented by silver crescent

Concerns: Pleasure, sexuality, vital force, unconscious emotions and desires

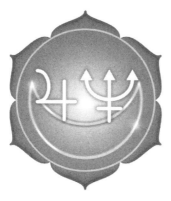

Fig. 2.24. Second, or sacral, chakra, Svadisthana

Sagittarean Astrology

Sagittarius is represented as a centaur archer, aiming his or her bow and arrow at a distant target. The arc is the flight path of the flaming arrow of our lives, upward to the peak and downward to the target. Sagittarius, the ninth sign of the natural zodiac and eleventh sign in the ATA, carries the numerical meanings of spiritual mastery, like the archer hitting the center of that distant target.

Sagittarius represents high idealism and wanting to make inclusive syntheses, such as in philosophy, education, history, law, and science. In myth, Chiron is the centaur on whom Sagittarius is based, a famous teacher of Greek heroes. It is said that Chiron believed in giving his students a well-rounded education. For example, a student might be studying philosophy but would also need to learn about the arts, physical development, science, martial arts, and other diverse subjects. Sagittarius likes the big picture and putting it all together into a meaningful whole. The centaur is part human and part horse. The human part represents the higher faculties, while the horse represents physical strength and endurance. Sagittarius presents an image of the balanced integration of human and horse—head in the stars and four fleet hooves on the ground.

The constellation of Sagittarius portrays the archer aiming his arrow toward the center of our Milky Way Galaxy. The sign Sagittarius, ruled by royal Jupiter, known as Zeus by the Greeks, contains the degree of the Galactic Center. Hence, Jupiter can be seen as the representative of the Galactic Center, a presence to uplift our solar system to a more expanded and aware level. In Vedic astrology, Jupiter is called the guru planet and has a spiritual presence and ability to teach the most profound lessons of enlightenment.

Since the sign and constellation Sagittarius contain the huge mass of our Galactic Center, it conveys the meaning of a much larger perspective. I like to think that the center of our Milky Way Galaxy is like the heart of a Great Mother Goddess, like Hera or Juno, and that the multitude of stars in this galaxy are the nurturing milk of her majestic logos. Jupiter entered his favorite sign of Sagittarius in 2018, transiting the Galactic Center, bringing a life-affirming and exalted boost in preparation for Jupiter's participation in the 2020 alignment in packed Capricorn and transition into the dawning of the New Age of Aquarius at the winter solstice of 2020.

Sagittarean Mythology

Chiron, the centaur in Greek myth, was the son of Cronus in his horse form. Chiron became known for kindness, wisdom, and justice and was a universal teacher. In addition to his expertise in traditional subjects of education, he was skilled in archery, like his friend Apollo, as well as in healing and the use of wild plants, a skill he learned from the goddess Artemis, another archer.

The sign Sagittarius, and especially the Sun in Sagittarius, is known to possess all of these traits of Chiron. The modern version of the story adds that the Sagittarian centaur can also be a party animal and an athlete; centaurs are friendly, outgoing, social, positive, high-minded, intelligent, and philosophical, to mention just a few of their many attributes.

Jupiter

Jupiter is the king of the gods and the planet of expansion and general good fortune. Beneficial Jupiter is the ruler of Sagittarius. Jupiter as the guru planet provides a wealth of spiritual abundance, with a natural ability for teaching and a sensitive attunement to many points of view. There are many stories about Jupiter/Zeus that demonstrate his power and his exuberance in pursuing sexual partners. As the ruler of Sagittarius, his wisdom is especially accented. In the Alchemical Tantric Arrangement, the placement of Sagittarius in this downward half of the zodiac reinforces the combination of physical strength and good mental abilities. This is especially useful in bringing the golden message of evolution gained from the highest chakras to a wide audience.

Juno

Astronomers believe that the asteroid belt between Mars and Jupiter was formed either when one large planet broke up or was unable to come together in its orbit due to King Jupiter's overpowering influence. Thus they have a special relationship to Jupiter, especially the four major asteroids: Ceres (now called a dwarf planet), Pallas Athene, Vesta, and Juno. In a similar fashion, mythologically speaking, the Greek and Roman gods Zeus and Jupiter represent the patriarchal perspective, overshadowing the matriarchal or gender-balanced perspective. Apparently, the patriarchy altered the myths, marrying formerly powerful and independent goddesses to gods in the new patriarchal dispensation.

As mentioned before, Juno/Hera was the queen of the divinities, royal mother, and wife. Both Juno and Jupiter are powerful representatives of Sagittarius. The asteroid Juno's aspects to Jupiter in the natal and Hermetic astrological charts can indicate either gender balance and cooperation or stress in relationships in general and in marriage specifically.

CAPRICORN

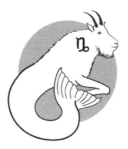

Ruling planet: Saturn
Associated asteroids: Juno, Chiron
Element: Earth
Quality: Cardinal
Numbers: Natural zodiac 10, Hermetic 12
Relative age: Elder
Gender: Feminine
Zodiac images: Goat with fish tail, mountain goat, unicorn
Body parts: Knees, skin, bones, teeth
Direction: South
Colors: Black, white, gray
Alchemical metal: Lead
Holidays: Christmas, New Year's Eve, Epiphany
Mythology: Saturn/Cronus, Chronos, Rhea, Juno/Hera, Pricus
Chakra: first, Muladhara (root support), base of the spine, anus
 Symbol: Red four-petaled lotus containing a golden square or cube
 Mantra: *Lang*
 Element: Earth
 Concerns: Food, resources, survival, safety, security, physical
 activity

Capricornian Astrology

Capricorn, as the tenth sign in the natural zodiac, is located at the top of the natural astrological chart, and, like the number 10, it symbolizes reaching for and attaining the highest goals. Beginning at the winter solstice in the Northern Hemisphere, Capricorn thereby represents

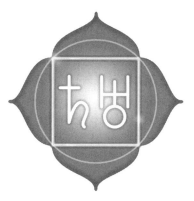

Fig. 2.25. First, or root, chakra, Muladhara

both the darkest time and the rebirth of the light—acknowledgment of renewal within a season of struggle. In Human Design, the first degree of Capricorn is related to the tenth hexagram of the I Ching, known as Treading on the Tail of the Tiger. This speaks to me of being experienced and wise enough to realize that it is best to stay alert and aware as we tread the karmically perilous journey of our lives. In the Human Design system, Capricorn gates are mostly placed in the first, or root, chakra, which is said to be like the gas tank that fuels the generator of the second chakra (see more about the Human Design system in chapter 4).

The lovely ringed planet Saturn is associated with Capricorn. Saturn is often pictured mythologically as an old man with a sickle, suggesting a harvest. Unlike the fruitful harvest of crops in autumn, this harvest occurs in deep winter and is of the more imperishable type: the soulful harvest of our actions in the world. Saturn is often considered a harsh influence but in truth simply delivers to us the karmic fruits of our long-term fateful labors, both delightful and depressing. He is karmically both the grim reaper and the glad reaper.

The sign Capricorn, being an earth sign, is known for being fortunate in terms of the material world and for qualities of conservation, painstaking discipline, and sensible effort. Capricorn is related to Chronos's wife, the Great Mountain Mother Rhea, and her daughter, Hera, who are goddesses of the rich and fertile Earth.

Rhea, the titanic mountain mother is perhaps a more easily approachable divinity than cosmic Chronos. Together, they are said to have reigned as king and queen of the golden age preceding the Olympian era. Cronus, the Greek name for Saturn, carries a connection to Chronos, the divinity of time. And indeed Saturn, being the most distant of the visible planets and therefore with the longest cycle, was used by the ancients to mark longer periods of time. Like the concept of time, Saturn as Chronos has some pretty heavy separation karma. Given the task of castrating his father, he cut apart the primal unity of his father and mother, Uranus and Gaia, which resulted in the separation of heaven from earth. This act became a pattern when emulated by his own son, Zeus/Jupiter, who eventually deposed him. Great Mother Rhea, on the other hand, played the role of protecting her children from these heavy patriarchal patterns. Rhea's daughter, Hera, like her mother, can be associated with the sign of Capricorn. Roman Juno, like Greek Hera, carries the archetype of the faithful wife and is the balance to wide-ranging Jupiter. Juno's connection to marriage fits conservative Capricorn, while her association with both partnership and art also puts her into alignment with the sign of balance, Libra, a sign where Saturn is exalted.

There is definitely a serious side to Capricorn; the sign is linked with our highest social goals and professions. Capricorn is thus the archetype of the true professor, one who professes and thus models the group's paramount ideals. Like the mountain goat, Capricorn stands balanced at life's peak.

Capricorn and the Longer Cycles

It is quite likely that we need to further contemplate the meaning of the sign Capricorn for our age. When the ancient Maya made the winter solstice of 2012 the end of their Long Count Calendar, I imagine they hoped to convey a special message to our modern age. The Capricorn Sun at the winter solstice of 2012 began its rise into the dark rift near the center of our Milky Way. Not only was this the midwinter of the year, but this occasion also marked for the Maya a cosmic midwinter point in the 26,000-year precession of the equinoxes and solstices. I envision the great horn of the goat as trumpeting a message from Galactic Central that these times, like treading on the tail of a tiger, require the time-tested wisdom, patience, care, and experience of our Capricorn leaders to pull us through these karmically perilous times. It would appear that we have been called to be some of these leaders. I can also easily imagine that, within each highly responsible adult Capricorn, there is a playful goat kid.

Saturn, ruler of Capricorn, entered his favorite sign at the end of 2017; however, 2020 was the year when Jupiter, Saturn, and several other planets came together with Pluto in this formidable sign. These amazing transits represent the dark night of the cycles, with Saturn's alchemical metal, lead, forming the container for the radioactive potential of Uranus and its metal, uranium, in the sign of the cupbearer, Aquarius. Jupiter and Saturn moved together into Aquarius at the end of 2020.

Capricornian Mythology

In myth, the constellation of Capricorn was placed in the sky by Zeus to commemorate Amalthea, the goat whose milk nourished baby Zeus. The word *Capricorn* means "goat horn." It is said that one of Amalthea's horns became the famous cornucopia, or horn of plenty.

In another Greek myth, Chronos was said to create the wise and talented fishgoat named Pricus, who lived near the seashore with his large family of fishgoats. The fishgoats would come ashore on occasion, but after some time on land, they tended to lose their higher faculties and became regular goats. This disturbed Pricus, especially after all of his family had lost their original mental and spiritual abilities, and he was left alone in the sea as the last true fishgoat.

Chronos, divinity of time, had given Pricus the talent of controlling time. So Pricus thought of the idea of turning back time to when all of his family of fishgoats were with him in the sea and had their former abilities. Alas, even after setting back time, his family of fishgoats continued to go ashore and become regular goats again, so the cycle was repeated over and over, with Pricus continuing to turn back the clock. Eventually, Pricus, tired of the sad situation, asked to give up his immortality. Then Chronos placed his image in the heavens as the constellation of Capricorn.

One profound interpretation of the story of Pricus is related to the idea of evolution. In the story of vast time periods, Pricus's dilemma is like our own in the sense that evolution from the sea to the land had both positive and negative consequences. Among many meanings, the cusp between Capricorn and Aquarius represents evolution, and the year 2020, when

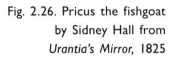

Fig. 2.26. Pricus the fishgoat
by Sidney Hall from
Urantia's Mirror, 1825

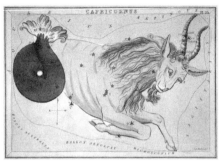

most of the Capricorn planetary stellium transitioned into Aquarius, represents the transformation from a fishgoat into a handsome cupbearer of ambrosia. What will we gain by this metamorphosis into immortal, brilliant light and what will we lose if the intelligence is artificial?

THE TURN OF THE WHEEL

This myth of Pricus is especially fitting for completing the journey through the signs and returning to the bottom of the Alchemical Tantric Arrangement of the zodiac. The story of the cycle of precession, and its likely relation to the great Hindu ages, or *yugas,* suggests a turning of the wheel of life, with its golden ups and dark downs of civilizations. Like the cycles of Pricus's generations, we can see evidence of golden ages in ancient Egypt and India, and the relative decadence of much of our present civilization.

Like Pricus, we might want to turn back time; however, unlike Pricus, we now know that there is another path (that is not really a path), represented by turning inward from the wheel of time to the timelessness and oneness held at the cusp between Capricorn and Aquarius, a point I have called the Chiron portal.

Leaving Capricorn brings us full circle back to the cusp of Aquarius and to a unique and profound understanding of the mythology of the signs and planets. As we continue to explore the richness of the Alchemical Tantric Arrangement we will find that it allows us to determine optimal astrological timing and symbolic appropriateness, which can give a greater depth to our understanding of the evolutionary path. Now that we have completed our journey through the zodiac, we turn our attention to the energy pathways of the Alchemical Tantric Arrangement.

3

The Serpent Kundalini, Energy Channels, and the Galactic Cross

The new shape of the zodiac in the Alchemical Tantric Arrangement mirrors the powerful tantric concepts of the kundalini serpent and the three energy channels, or nadis, which spiral through the chakras. We will also explore the powerful symbolism of the Galactic Cross and its connection with the equinoxes and the solstices.

THE SERPENT KUNDALINI

Kundalini is a key part of tantric yoga and is inextricably linked with the chakras. This subtle energy visualized as a coiled snake is located at the base of the spine in the Muladhara, or root, chakra. When awakened naturally or through various yogic practices, the kundalini energy is said to uncoil and travel upward through the seven chakras on intertwining energy pathways or channels called nadi. The three principal nadis are the feminine ida nadi, the masculine pingala nadi, and the central sushumna nadi.

In the tantric yoga system, this awakened energy provides profound knowledge and abilities that help the practitioner to evolve. Generally, it is assumed that individuals evolve in many ways—physically, mentally, psychologically, spiritually, and so on—via the lessons of their life experiences, either at a natural pace or, more efficiently, with the help of specialized knowledge and practices, such as those of yoga. The phrase *kundalini rising* refers to the accelerated pace of human evolution.

Volumes could be written about the rich symbolism of the serpent, an image whose meaning ranges all the way from evil to divine. For many reasons, but perhaps especially due to their long shape and a tendency to appear out of holes in the ground, snakes have been associated in myth and symbol with lengths of time and space, and especially the upward movement of energy. The snake or serpent's many attributes produce an overall image of a creature that carries a mysterious power or knowledge. See the books *The Cosmic Serpent: DNA and the Origins of Knowledge* by Jeremy Narby and *Serpent in the Sky: The High Wisdom of Ancient Egypt* by John Anthony West, two very illuminating books among thousands demonstrating the amazingly suggestive connections among the images of the serpent in myth, yoga, shamanism, and religions worldwide.

The vast body of knowledge concerning the cosmic serpent contains a very clear hint that the serpent and related dragon are often pointing toward a powerful evolutionary energy that is also represented by the serpentine DNA molecule and the *siddhis,* or paranormal powers of yoga, which are more fully explored later in chapter 9.

THE THREE NADIS AND THE ALCHEMICAL TANTRIC ARRANGEMENT

The zodiac arranged according to the ATA relates the circle of astrological signs and the seven chakras to the three primary subtle nerves, the ida, pingala, and sushumna, in this way:

Ida, the tantric name of the channel of the cooling lunar breath, shown in figure 3.1 by the upward-moving silver serpent; pingala, the heating solar channel shown by the downward-moving golden serpent; and the central evolutionary channel named sushumna, passageway for the evolutionary energy, or shakti, which is likened to the powerful serpent named kundalini.

Pingala
(golden downward serpent)

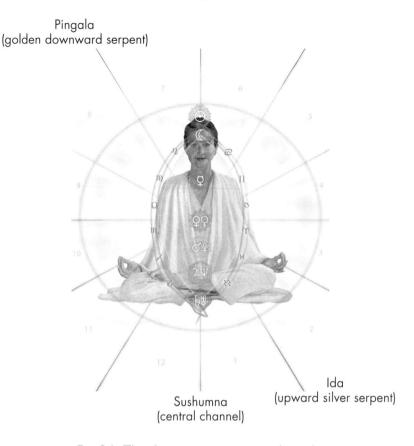

Ida
(upward silver serpent)

Sushumna
(central channel)

Fig. 3.1. The three primary energy channels:
ida, pingala, and sushumna

As will be more thoroughly illustrated below, the process of transforming consciousness, symbolized by the movement through the alchemical metals from lead to gold and the raising of the kundalini serpent energy, adds new and important understandings to the progression through the signs of the zodiac. The order of zodiac signs, alternating between feminine and masculine, correlates with the two intertwining serpents of energy moving up and down the chakras, similar to the two serpents wrapped around the central rod of Hermes's staff, the caduceus. This connection to Hermes and the Western Hermetic tradition is why the Alchemical Tantric Arrangement, when applied and used practically, can also be known as Hermetic Astrology.

THE GALACTIC CROSS
AND THE GALACTIC CENTER

Precession: this is a big idea that starts with a very basic observation. We all know the Earth spins on its axis, causing the turning of the day.

But a more profound and unfamiliar cycle is the very large one that results from the Earth's wobble, like a spinning top, which takes around 26,000 years to make a full circle. At times, the axis of the poles is inclined more or less toward the Galactic Center of the Milky Way. This wobble causes the equinoxes and solstices to shift 1 degree every 72 years relative to the stars and constellations, giving us twelve 2150+ year "ages" such as the Age of Pisces and the Age of Aquarius. In western tropical astrology the two equinoxes and the two solstices begin with the four cardinal signs, Aries, Cancer, Libra, and Capricorn. Connecting these four signs creates a cross in the wheel of the year as well as the grand wheel of galactic precession, vital for astrological orientation. It is clear that many ancient cultures knew of the great cycle of precession and gave very high importance to it. The grand square, or cross, in the astrological chart, and especially the cardinal cross, has symbolic resonance with the great cycle of precession. This resonance will help us to better comprehend the vast power of the four primary directions of the Alchemical Tantric Arrangement of the zodiac.

In astrology it is assumed that alignments of planets to other planets and to other celestial phenomena result in the sharing of information among them. Important alignments to the Galactic Center, therefore, can be seen as communications, with energy pulses or vibrations radiating out from the center of our galaxy, perhaps carrying important information to our Sun and thence to the Earth.

The Four Signs of the Great Cross

A special connection between the Galactic Center and the great cross of the Earth's equinoxes and solstices can be seen in the astrological glyphs for the four cardinal signs.

Capricorn. The goat with a fish tail. The goat horn is a musical instrument, trumpeting vibrating sound waves from the great heavenly sea. (The heavens are often viewed as oceanic, hence Capricorn's fish tail.) Capricorn's cornucopia is the corn or horn of plenty. Capricorn's fish tail, like the sea serpent, connects us to the rich symbolism of the snake, which moves wave-like and river-like. The serpent also conjures an image of the spiraling twin snakes of the DNA, molecule of the inner galaxy, and kundalini, the tantric yoga serpent of accelerated evolution.

Cancer. This glyph can also be viewed as a spiral galaxy. Cancer, ruling the breasts, suggests the Milky Way and the Galactic Center (as noted earlier, *gala* is the Greek word for "milk"). Cancer is the sign also associated with the stomach and nurturance, like the Galactic Center electromagnetically feeding her stars and planets.

Aries. The ram's cosmically spiral horn is blown as a spiritual musical instrument, quite possibly with vibrations in tune with the Galactic Center. The ram's horn trumpet is still used in Jewish religious ceremonies.

Libra. The sign of the scale and of balance has a glyph that looks like a spiral galaxy viewed from the side with its central bulge.

The Alchemical Tantric Arrangement of the signs puts a special emphasis on the cross-quarter times of mid-Aquarius and mid-Leo. These subtle transition times are halfway between the solstices and equinoxes. Cross-quarter times are actually the beginning points of the four seasons rather than the solstices and equinoxes, which are the midpoints of the seasons (see the section that follows, "The Four New Years"). They are especially important since they can alert us to the major thresholds at the end of summer and winter. Mid-Leo is the subtle beginning of autumn, and mid-Aquarius is the subtle beginning of spring (in the Northern Hemisphere). Chinese New Year, in February, marks this subtle shift at the time of the Aquarius new Moon. The dragon masks and firecrackers during the celebration of Chinese New Year emphasize this passage as a spiritual time for the awakening of primal energies!

THE FOUR NEW YEARS

For a more complete understanding of the Alchemical Tantric Arrangement, it is instructive to look now at the four major New Years because the important portal on the cusp between Capricorn and Aquarius is located near three of these times.

1. New Year based on the winter solstice point (in the Northern Hemisphere)
2. New Year beginning on January 1
3. Chinese New Year, based on the beginning of spring in the Northern Hemisphere
4. New Year based on the beginning of the first sign, Aries, in the natural order of the zodiac at the spring equinox

These four times comprise a progression in subtlety.

Winter solstice in the Northern Hemisphere can be considered the first and most subtle starting point of the New Year, although occurring near the end of the old calendar year. As the southernmost point in the Sun's cycle, it accents the return of the light from this darkest time, the center of winter. Winter solstice makes a good beginning for the New Year because of its proximity to Christmas and its association with divine birth.

New Year in the Western calendar occurs at the first instant after midnight between December 31 and January 1, so the astrological chart for this popular beginning time will always show the Sun near the nadir (lowest point in the astrological chart) at around 10 degrees of Capricorn. (Capricorn has an affinity with the number 10.) Fortunately, this makes Libra the rising sign each year, and therefore Venus the overall ruler of these calendar New Year charts. Looking at the symbolism of midnight, close to midwinter in the Northern Hemisphere, this version of the New Year also accents the return of the light from a period of darkness.

I have named this point around 10 degrees of Capricorn the

Morpheus point, after the Roman divinity of sleep and dreams. Morpheus is a shape-shifter and carries some of the flavor of the New Year's Eve masquerade ball, which also emphasizes Venus, since the custom is to kiss the person you are with at the exact beginning of the New Year. I have found it instructive to watch the transits over this Morpheus point each year. Roughly between the years of 2011 and 2014, Pluto, fittingly the divinity of the underworld, had been transiting the bottom of the chart and thereby coloring each New Year's chart with the apocalyptic symbolism of Hades and Persephone.

Serious Saturn's presence near the Morpheus point in 2018 and 2019 added an extra weight to the bottom of the New Year charts in this period. Capricorn's rulership by Saturn, and this consequential sign's connection to the alchemical metal lead and to the first, or root, chakra, produces a heavy and grounding symbolism. The name of the twelfth month, December, once again emphasizes the number 10; the name comes from the Latin word *decem,* meaning "ten," because it was originally the tenth month of the year.

The month of January brings the mythic presence of the Roman two-faced divinity Janus, looking back over the past year and forward to the new year. At the end of 2017, Saturn entered Capricorn and, in 2018 and 2019, transited the Morpheus point. Jupiter did the same at the beginning of 2020. It is instructive to compare the effects of all the planets that transit the Morpheus point, but especially recently transiting Pluto, Saturn, and Jupiter.

Chinese New Year, sometimes called Lunar New Year, marks the early stirrings of spring, during the first cross-quarter time after the winter solstice. In the Western Hemisphere, it is based on the new Moon of Aquarius, so that both the Sun and the Moon are at the beginning of their cycles, although it is often shown on the Western calendar for the next day referring to the time zone difference in China. This New Year resonates with Aquarius and the first, or root, chakra, which begins the upward, accumulating path of the Alchemical Tantric Arrangement.

The Spring Equinox occurs at the first degree of Aries and marks the center of the spring season. Starting the year at this point is also fitting in terms of the upward, accumulating path of the ATA. Fiery Aries is the first and foremost natural sign, being the cardinal sign of fire and related to the direction of the great eastern Sun. Aries is followed by earthy Vacca/Taurus, most fixed of the fixed signs, which in turn is followed by the most mutable of the mutable signs, airy Gemini, and then another cardinal sign, watery Cancer. Thus, on our way to the royal sign Leo, associated with the uppermost crown chakra, we will have passed through the four most archetypical elemental signs: fire, earth, air, and water.

This is the fourth time of beginning a New Year and sometimes is called the beginning of the season (spring in the Northern Hemisphere) for those who are not looking for subtle signs. Looking at all four of these New Years offers a wide view of the coming year. It was especially instructive for the year 2020, which had many important planets transiting the vital portal between Capricorn and Aquarius.

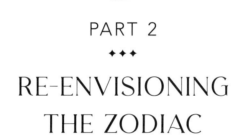

PART 2

✦✦✦

RE-ENVISIONING THE ZODIAC

Working with the Alchemical Tantric Arrangement

4

The New Meaning of Hermetic Astrology

In part 1 we saw a new order in the traditional planetary rulers of the twelve signs. Another key to the Alchemical Tantric Arrangement comes when we examine the alchemical metals associated with these ruling planets. Just as the signs share a planetary ruler, they also share the associated metal for that ruler (see figure 4.1).

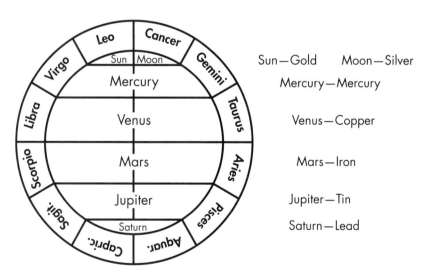

Fig. 4.1. The alchemical arrangement of the signs with their planetary rulers and associated alchemical metals

Image from *Galactic Alignment* by John Major Jenkins.

Therefore, in a manner similar to "translating" the original Rosetta Stone, we have accomplished the first step in our process of translation by creating the alchemical arrangement of the signs. This arrangement puts Saturn and its alchemical metal, lead, at the bottom of the chart and the Sun and its alchemical metal, gold, at the top. The resulting order reflects the understanding of alchemy as the process of transforming lead into gold.

Medieval alchemy acknowledged a correlation between planets in the heavens and metals in the earth: as above, so below. In fact, alchemy used the very same symbols for both metals and planets, as shown in figure 4.2.

ALCHEMICAL SYMBOLS

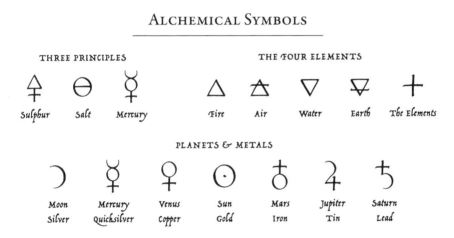

Fig. 4.2. Alchemical symbols of planets and metals

Alchemy's goal of transforming lead into gold, in a profound sense, is a metaphor for the transformation of consciousness. We can see in the progression of the metals from gray lead, to useful tin and iron, to beautiful copper, shiny silver, and glistening gold, a movement toward more beauty and value. Likewise, the goal of the spiritual path is the transformation of consciousness from more conditioned patterns of thinking and behavior to freedom and enlightenment.

ADDING THE TANTRIC CONNECTION

The seven traditional planets and their seven alchemical metals now correspond perfectly to the seven chakras of tantric yoga:

Lead and Saturn give a cool neutral gray density to the first, or root, chakra.

Tin and Jupiter suggest shine and malleability to the second, or sacral, chakra.

Iron and Mars bring hardness, strength, and weaponry to the third, or navel, chakra.

Copper and Venus convey beauty and conductivity to the fourth, or heart, chakra.

Mercury, metal and planet, convey shiny movement to the fifth, or throat, chakra.

Silver and the Moon suggest cool radiant beauty and value to the sixth, or brow, chakra.

Gold and the Sun offer rich warm value and radiance to the seventh, or crown, chakra.

The relationship between astrology and the chakra system has been and continues to be of interest to many practitioners of both yoga and astrology. This powerful and illuminating relationship is thereby established.

The first version of the Alchemical Tantric Arrangement (ATA) shown in figure 4.3 is taken from *Conscious Conception: Elemental Journey through the Labyrinth of Sexuality,* which my former wife, Jeannine Parvati, and I published in 1986, after several years of preparation. In this book, we wrote about astrology in terms of consciously conceiving, and it was in this book that I presented my first version or vision of the ATA. This first version is a rather crude rendering of astrology's Rosetta Stone (figure 4.3), while figure 4.4 is the current version. Both images demonstrate the integration of all three languages of the astrological Rosetta Stone: astrology, alchemy, and

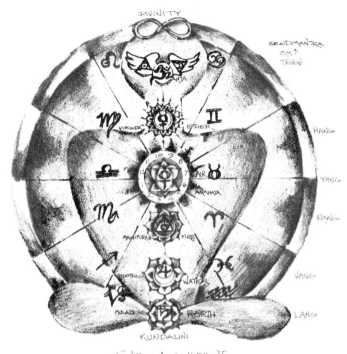

Fig. 4.3. The first Alchemical Tantric Arrangement

the tantric chakra system. In both figures, the tantric chakra system has been overlaid onto the ATA. The seven planetary metals correlate with the seven chakras, from lead at the bottom, or root chakra, to gold at the top, or crown chakra. Importantly, the overlay creates a perfect correlation between the central heart chakra's twelve petals, the twelve signs of the zodiac, and the twelve houses of astrology. The heart chakra is central to the chakra system with three chakras above and three below, and its symbol is a six-pointed star of two interlocking triangles pointing up and down. Thus, in the ATA (fig. 4.4) the center of the chakra system is perfectly aligned with the central point of the astrology chart.

Beginning with Capricorn and Aquarius on the bottom of the zodiac wheel (relating to the first chakra), note that both of these signs were traditionally ruled by Saturn, whose metal is lead in alchemy, also

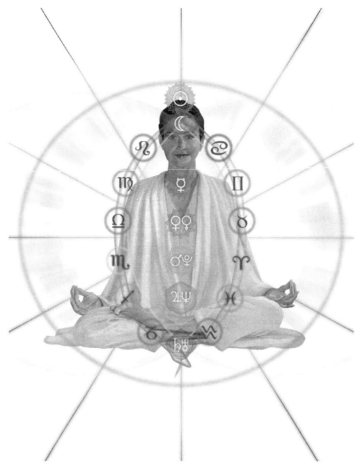

Fig. 4.4. The latest version of
the Alchemical Tantric Arrangement

known as the prima materia, or the primary material, of the alchemical process of transformation. Moving upward, the next pairs of signs are Sagittarius and Pisces, ruled by Jupiter (alchemical metal tin, second chakra); Scorpio and Aries, ruled by Mars (iron, third chakra); Libra and Vacca/Taurus, ruled by Venus (copper, fourth chakra); Virgo and Gemini, ruled by Mercury (mercury, fifth chakra); Cancer, ruled by the Moon (silver, sixth chakra); and finally Leo, ruled by the golden Sun and related to the seventh chakra, or the thousand-petaled lotus crown chakra.

This arrangement symbolizes what the alchemists called the philosopher's stone, a tool with the legendary alchemical ability to transform lead into gold. Similarly, in the chakra system, the movement upward through the chakras follows the awakening of a powerful transformative energy called kundalini and its movement through the seven chakras and their five associated subtle elements (earth, water, fire, air, and ether) and two super-subtle elements (sound and light).

TABLE OF CORRESPONDENCES

CHAKRA	SIGNS	TRADITIONAL RULER, ALCHEMICAL METAL	NEW RULER, ALCHEMICAL METAL
First	Aquarius, Capricorn	Saturn, Lead	Uranus, Uranium
Second	Pisces, Sagittarius	Jupiter, Tin	Neptune, Neptunium
Third	Scorpio, Aries	Mars, Iron	Pluto, Plutonium
Fourth	Vacca/Taurus, Libra	Venus, Copper	Eris, Americium

TRANSITING THROUGH THE ALCHEMICAL TANTRIC ARRANGEMENT

Of primary value is pondering the movement of planets or their transits through the cycle of the ATA or Hermetic arrangement of the zodiac. Knowing the signs and their association with the two directions of the chakras, those who are acquainted with transits can now use astrology to tune into the most appropriate times for their meditations and actions. For example, in 2020, there was a major alignment of planets, including the solar system heavyweights, Jupiter and Saturn, meeting apocalyptic Pluto in Capricorn near the bottom of the ATA. At the end of 2020, Jupiter and Saturn entered Aquarius and soon thereafter began their movement upward through the cosmic chakra system. According to the ATA system, several influential planetary cycles, especially Pluto, Saturn, and Jupiter, dipped into the darkest part of their cycles before turning upward again. The transition of these significant planets from downward Capricorn into upward Aquarius was an excellent time to focus on awakening kundalini while the cosmic energy was at this pivotal point. The effect on the whole Earth in 2020, associated with these major transits of this highly charged area of the Hermetic chart, was truly astounding!

Recalling that the Mayan Long Count Calendar ended exactly on the winter solstice of 2012, the significant planetary events mentioned above point toward a similar image—a dark period of the Kali Yuga. Although foreboding in some sense, it is also an auspicious time to meditate in tune with the planets, aligning with the symbolism of the rebirth of the light following a period of intense darkness.

THE HUMAN DESIGN SYSTEM

Since the publication of *Conscious Conception* in 1986, I have been slowly refining my vision of the ATA, with the help of tracking the major Capricorn formations, including the cardinal grand crosses and the Mayan Long Count Calendar end date at the winter solstice of 2012, as outlined above.

A significant influence on this new vision of astrology was a system called Human Design, conceived by Ra Uru Hu, a Canadian astrologer formerly called Alan Krakower. Similar to my unusual experience on the island of Formentera in 1973, Ra had an interesting experience on a Spanish island named Ibiza near Formentera. His experience lasted about a week during the winter just after New Year 1987, and he seemingly received information on how astrology, yoga, and several other systems could be synthesized. The Human Design system integrates parts of several traditions including astrology, the chakra system (with nine primary chakras), the I Ching, the kabbalistic Tree of Life, and acupuncture channels. There is considerable overlap between the Human Design system and the Hermetic astrology of the ATA.

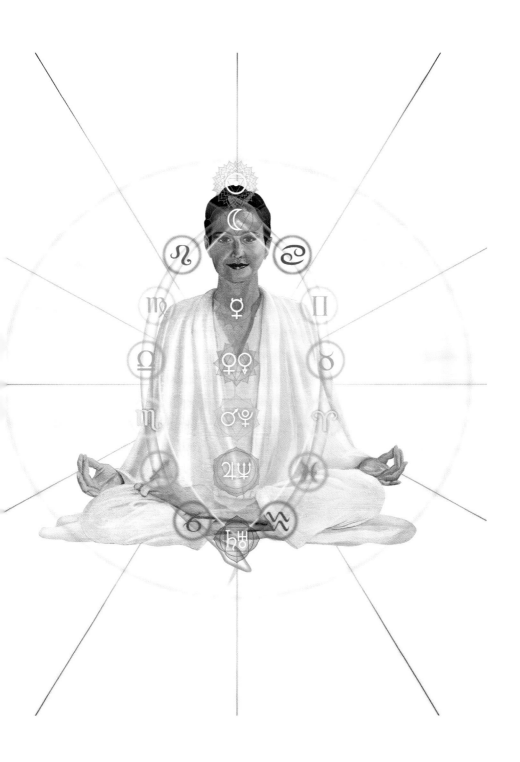

Plate 1. The Alchemical Tantric Arrangement. Note that the zodiac symbols are presented in the color of their corresponding chakra.

CHAKRA CORRESPONDENCE

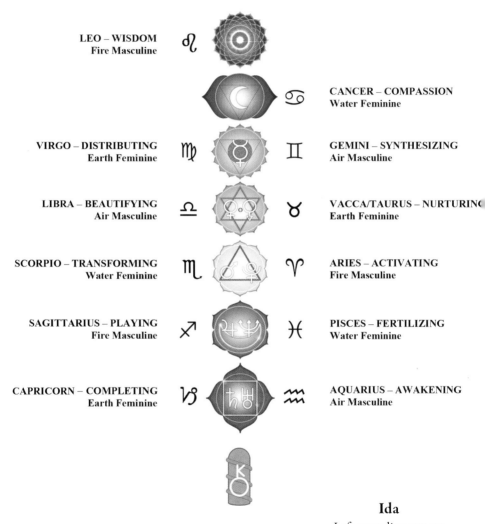

Pingala
Right descending serpent
spiraling down via masculine signs

Right Nostril   Left Nostril

LEO – WISDOM
Fire Masculine

CANCER – COMPASSION
Water Feminine

VIRGO – DISTRIBUTING
Earth Feminine

GEMINI – SYNTHESIZING
Air Masculine

LIBRA – BEAUTIFYING
Air Masculine

VACCA/TAURUS – NURTURING
Earth Feminine

SCORPIO – TRANSFORMING
Water Feminine

ARIES – ACTIVATING
Fire Masculine

SAGITTARIUS – PLAYING
Fire Masculine

PISCES – FERTILIZING
Water Feminine

CAPRICORN – COMPLETING
Earth Feminine

AQUARIUS – AWAKENING
Air Masculine

Ida
Left ascending serpent
spiraling upward via feminine signs

Plate 2. Chakras, their associated zodiac signs, and Hermetic keywords.
Note the two serpents spiraling up through feminine (Earth and Water)
and descending through masculine (Fire and Air) signs.

Teachers of Human Design have come into my life on several occasions, and I find it intriguing how Human Design has paralleled my development of the ATA. When one looks at the distribution of zodiac signs in the nine chakras of the Human Design bodygraph, it tends generally to follow the alchemical progression of the ATA upward from Capricorn-Aquarius in the root center. I think that the ATA presented in my book, developed after more than forty years of incubation, could be especially helpful to practitioners of Human Design and vice versa. I intuit that many profound ancient systems are based on an understanding of what modern science calls the DNA molecule; and, of course, the I Ching has a strong resonance with DNA (see the provocative book *DNA and the I Ching* by Johnson F. Yan).

5
Astrological Chakra Symbolism

We have demonstrated an expansion of the meaning of the twelve signs of the zodiac and their ruling planets by the addition of the seven chakras. We turn now to an expansion of the meaning of the chakras through their association with the signs of the zodiac and their ruling planets.

THE CHAKRAS AND THEIR ASSOCIATED ZODIAC SIGNS AND PLANETS

First, Root, Chakra:
Capricorn, Aquarius, Saturn, and Uranus

The first chakra is known as the root chakra. The Muladhara lotus, or root chakra mandala, is a symbol of the blossoming of the apparent everything from the central dot, bindu, or flower bud. This dimensionless dot represents the white hole into the void of no-thing, which is the womb of everything. It is timeless and without location, so it is not born and does not die; there is no place else to go. There is no inside or outside.

Capricorn, as the most mature of the earth signs, represents a full cycle of grounded experience. Aquarius brings the awakening energy of spring and the initiation of a new cycle and new age. Capricorn and Aquarius form a semisextile aspect. (See chapter 11 for the meaning of aspects.) The primal or root duality of the planets Saturn and Uranus strongly influence the meaning of the Muladhara chakra. The meeting of Saturn, representing conservation, and Uranus, representing innovation, in this chakra involves an important shift from the downward-distributing channel (pingala) to the upward accumulating channel (ida).

The cupbearer's drink of ambrosia that brought immortality to the divinities represents the wisdom of nonduality, which is just "this, as it is." A drink from this cup results in the imaginary death of that which has never been—the separate self. This is the true dawning of the Age of Aquarius—absolute freedom, for no separate one.

Second Chakra:
Sagittarius, Pisces, Jupiter, and Neptune

The second chakra, the sacral chakra, is one of primal duality/ nonduality. It is tenderly represented by the lovers, who are always exchanging thoughts, smells, breath, and fluids. They are not separate, and their intercourse is a statement of the apparent dance of the one and the two or, perhaps better, the zero and the one.

Sagittarius, a sign of both wisdom and celebration, contributes the centaur's diverse qualities such as being both a teacher and party animal. Pisces offers a mystical feminine depth and the rich symbolism of the sea: foggy, clear, calm, stormy, vast, overwhelming, and the destination of rivers. Sagittarius and Pisces form a square aspect (see chapter 11). Their ruling planets, Jupiter and Neptune, embody the vastness of the sky and sea. Both these signs represent the synthesis of opposites: human with animal and land with sea.

Wave and water, ocean and river. It is all apparent movement of the same nonstuff. There are no things separate from this. Every "thing" that is happening is not happening to any separate one, especially not "me." The lotus of the second sacral chakra is the second mandala and therefore another diagram of the union of the every-thing and the no-thing.

Third Chakra:
Scorpio, Aries, Mars, and Pluto

The Manipura lotus, or navel chakra, is another diagram of always already existing oneness. It is a mandala of the jeweled city, located at the prenatal center navel, reminding us of our original and always connection to the Great Primal Mother. It is the center of the powerful awakening to the emptiness. Its mantra, *om mani padme hung* ("oh jewel in the lotus"), evokes the mandala of the jewel in the center of the lotus. The jewel is the Buddha or awakened one who realizes that there is nothing to attain and no separate self to attain anything. *Form is emptiness, and emptiness is form.* The word *emptiness* is likewise empty, as are all these words. The map is not the territory, and the territory is not the territory.

Scorpio brings an aura of mystery, of death, and of the powerful manipulation of energy. Aries gives this chakra even more emphasis on fiery yang activism. Scorpio and Aries form the 150 degree inconjunct or quincunx aspect, an angle that I have come to know as alchemical. (See chapter 11.) Containing both the square and the sextile (90 + 60 = 150), it has both the challenge and the ability, creating an evolutionary opportunity. If Mars is fire, Pluto is radioactive fire, and their intensity adds the imaginal underworld of Hades's realm to the mix. Fire and radioactive fire are the images of power and radical transformation.

Fourth Chakra:
Libra, Vacca/Taurus, Venus, and Eris

The fourth chakra, or Anahata lotus of the heart chakra, puts the emphasis on the central and unmoving axis around which all the great wheels revolve. Realizing the empty fullness represented by the mandala of two intersecting triangles of up and down, in and out, female and male, we see their nonsubstantial relational unity. It's much ado about nothing, a golden apple thrown into the ego party. In this unity there is no place to go, nothing to get, and no one to get anything. This is the center of unconditional love that is born of the peace of the absolute perfection of what is. After all the busy cycles on the wheels of apparent life, this is the calm restful center, the heart center. *Anahata* ("unstruck sound") is the sound of one hand clapping, the unified love that passes all understanding

Libra brings balance, harmony, grace in relationships, and artistic gifts. Vacca/Taurus conveys an aura of fertility, sensuality, and feminine charm. Libra and Vacca/Taurus form an inconjunct or quincunx aspect. Venus and Eris are a pair that can be counted on to make a dramatic influence on the fourth chakra's party.

Fifth Chakra:
Gemini, Virgo, Mercury
The fifth chakra is located in the region of the throat, making it a link between the body and the head, the heart and the mind. The mandala of the fifth chakra is a blue-green lotus with sixteen petals containing a circle or sphere of many sparkling shades of blue, suggesting the ephemeral quality of ether, or space. It conveys the spaciousness of nonduality.

Virgo carries the image of a powerful goddess of healing and of the harvest, crystal clarity, and precision. Gemini contributes wily wisdom, curiosity, exploration, and synthesis. Virgo and Gemini form a square aspect. Mercury is the guide and connector. Mercury as the moveable metal and messenger for the divinities is symbolic of bridging gaps and connecting realms. A key alchemical goal is the integration of the various dichotomies such as up and down, right and left, female and male, earth and heaven. Hermes/Mercury makes it one.

Sixth Chakra:
Cancer, Moon
The sixth chakra is the brow, or Ajna (authority or command), chakra and has strong spiritual connotations represented by the two light-blue or white petals of primal duality and the full Moon of enlightenment behind the symbol for the powerful universal mantra *Om*. This mantra is the sound of creation and before.

Homey Cancer and the cool feminine Moon add a royal compassionate aura yet still with great power. Cancer lends an aura of the queen mother's presence and lunar luminosity to the chakra of the third eye. I have often pondered the meaning of ultra-feminine Cancer as the sign at the bright summer solstice. It was not until I fully witnessed the full Cancer Moon at the highest (most northern) point in the sky, that I realized her beautiful yet powerful majesty. She is the female commander of the night sky.

Seventh Chakra:
Leo, Sun

The highest chakra is the crown chakra, and is connected to the highest of celestial bodies, the Sun. This chakra, viewed as the highest mandala of one thousand petals of all colors, is pointing downward, suggesting the unity of completion and return. The seed sound is silent and the Om is of light.

Leo presents the royal solar radiance and magnificence. Cancer and Leo form a semisextile aspect, their union is expressed in many ways including the sound and light of Om as two sides of the same coin of silver and gold. The Sun, of course, is the star of our planetary system and the metaphor of stardom fits not only with Leo's dramatic presence but also the royal crown chakra at the top of the head. The Sun as center of the crown mandala has a dot in the center that emphasizes the timeless and dimensionless final goal—the empty fullness of the journey and its completion. Note that this final chakra fits the top of the skull and is pointing downward; therefore, it is like a cup pouring out its contents of ambrosia—distributing nourishment for the return journey.

Who is pouring the cup of ambrosia? Who is receiving it?

The rising of kundalini energy is especially active in the upper three chakras, and as mandalas they are each equally complete in themselves; they create another threefold section emphasizing the triangle of the divine couple and the minister presiding over their marriage—Sun, Moon, and Mercury.

I have noted the following divisions in the seven chakras based on number:

One central heart chakra.

Two chakras at the base of the spine focus on the male lingam and female flower, and two chakras in the head focus on the marriage of Sun and Moon.

Three chakras leading upward into union from Mercury in Gemini to Moon and Sun and then another triangle of three distributing the energy of the golden union of Moon and Sun via Mercury down again into Virgo.

Four radioactive chakras ruled by Uranus, Neptune, Pluto, and Eris.

Five subtle elements lead from Virgo's element of space down to Capricorn's earth.

HERMETIC JOURNEY THROUGH THE TWELVEFOLD SIGNS

One important contribution of the ATA is that the cycle of the twelve signs can be meaningfully divided into the *seven upward-moving signs from Aquarius to Leo,* related to the seven ascending chakras, and the *five descending signs from Virgo to Capricorn,* which emphasize the return through the chakras to the root center related to the five elements. This complete twelvefold cycle demonstrates that the spiritual path is not simply an ascent into the upper subtle centers but a cycle that includes a sharing of the alchemical harvest and a return to the vital roots. Like inhalation and exhalation, both the journey up the chakras and down are vital. Although we tend to emphasize the ascent to the higher chakras, the lower chakras are especially related in the human body to elimination, and extremely important to health. The first four chakras, related to the primal elements are also important for eliminating feces (earth), urine (water), sweat via the skin (fire), and breath (air).

Aquarius and the First Chakra

Aquarius, with its flowing ambrosia, the drink of immortality, suggests transcendence of the primal human condition. A related symbol is the Tree of Life, which bears golden fruit of immortality. The Tree of Life, with roots deep into the earth and branches reaching heavenward, resembles the tree-shaped subtle body of the chakras and nadis. The Tree of Life is often shown with a resident protective dragon or serpent wrapped around it, symbolically linked with the coiled energy of the serpent kundalini, which, in the tantric chakra system, is said to be resting coiled around a phallic lingam until it springs upward after being awakened.

The emphasis is on the subtle awakenings of spring, represented by Groundhog Day; the not-so-subtle awakening power of surprising Uranus and its alchemical metal, uranium; and the love energy of St. Valentine. These facets, taken together, make Aquarius the perfect sign to begin the alchemical, tantric path. Think of the preceding sign, Capricorn, as the time of winter's snow-covered frozen earth and Aquarius as bringer of the first stirrings of spring, when tender but hardy green sprouts start reaching upward through the snow to the crisp, cool blue air above.

Aquarius is primarily about the energy of springing forth; its key Hermetic word is *awakening*. There is more than a hint of sexual metaphor as the kundalini serpent has similarities to the spermatozoa ejaculated from the lingam. Kundalini could also symbolize sublimating sexual energy. Both the natural movement toward reproduction and the turn inward toward absolute union are represented in this sign of the cupbearer.

Pisces and the Second Chakra

The crescent Moon shown in the second chakra is like a cup, chalice, or arc, all suggestive of the womb. The ovum-like Moon is especially resonant with watery Pisces, as are the multitude of fish-like sperm. The sign of Pisces is at home in the waters of the sexual second chakra. Oceanic Neptune, his partner Salacia, and his fertile brother, Jupiter/Zeus, are all well suited for this sign and chakra.

All three water signs, Scorpio, Cancer, and Pisces, make a good match for this sexual second chakra; however, boundary-dissolving Pisces is the most resonant, in my opinion. Scorpio's association with death and power and Cancer's motherly qualities place them second and third to Pisces for vast oceanic enjoyment of flowing together in sexual union.

The key Hermetic word for Pisces is *fertilizing*.

Aries and the Third Chakra

The third chakra being related to the element of fire, fiery Aries is appropriate here. There is a resonance of the sign Aries and its ruler Mars with the navel area and the digestive fire within. Aries has a passionate hunger for intensity that can become assertive and even aggressive.

The key Hermetic word for Aries is *activating*. Mars/Ares is the warrior god; while sacrifice is a vital part of being a warrior, being active in general is fundamental to his nature. In this upward, accumulating side of the Hermetic arrangement of the signs, Aries plays the vigorous role of forging ahead, going boldly into life's turmoil. The equilibrium of the equinox, found at the beginning of Aries's sign, is symbolized in the ram's two horns. His headstrong energy is ready to break through all blocks. Fire and fury have their place in a spiritual warrior; Aries together with the third chakra can constellate the hero and heroine archetype.

Vacca/Taurus and the Fourth Chakra

Moving up the kundalini ladder, we come to the fourth and central heart center of the chakra system, with three chakras below and three above. Here, we encounter the six-pointed star, composed of two interlocking triangles, symbolic of union in general and of the marriage of the spiritual and the material. This central chakra is also the center of the astrological mandala. The heart chakra's twelve petals correspond to the twelve houses and twelve signs. This is a pivotal center as part of the upward progression of the signs and also it is the ultimate central bindu: love is the key.

The Hermetic phrase for Vacca/Taurus is *nurturing*. Although love is central, there is a wide continuum among the various meanings of the word. Both rulers of Vacca/Taurus, Venus and Eris, have their wonderful and problematic sides. The two signs related to Venus and Eris in the Alchemical Tantric Arrangement of the signs of the zodiac, Libra and Vacca/Taurus, represent the duality of harmony and strife. As noted earlier in part 1, the Judgment of Paris features Eris and her golden apple of contention. Paris, ordered by Zeus to choose among three powerful goddesses, can represent our human dilemma. We are also confronted by our own difficult choices concerning these three great earth goddesses—the maiden, represented by Venus/Aphrodite; the wife and mother, represented by Hera; and the Crone, represented by Athene—and their respective attributes of passion, responsibility, and wisdom. Paris's quandary, like all of ours, is to find the emphasis or balance that best fits our particular life's situation. Astrology can guide us on our journey through love's labyrinth to help us unpack the promise and the dilemma that Paris had to meet in choosing among these three great earth goddesses.

If the problematic parts of love illustrated in the myth of the golden apple are resolved, then we might be able to rise to the higher octave of unconditional love. The nondual description of the absolute as *satchitananda,* which might be translated as "being" (*sat*), "consciousness" (*chit*), and "bliss" (*ananda*), or life-light-love, suggests that consciousness and unconditional love are inherent in everything. Perhaps we get a taste of this kind of love when we fall (or rise!) in love, and all the world glows in the bliss of perfection—until the mind gets involved, that is.

Gemini and the Fifth Chakra

Since Gemini is a mutable air sign and therefore like the changeable mind, it fits well with this fifth chakra of the subtle element—ether, or space. Like Gemini's ruling planet, Mercury, messenger of the divinities, speech, and expression are also highlighted in this fifth chakra, which is located in the area of the throat. The upward-accumulating half of the zodiac, which we are metaphorically ascending, can be viewed as developing the traits necessary to make the very best use of the pinnacle, or zenith, of the chart. This might be called the process of enlightenment or unification.

With the sign Gemini, there is a reaching upward toward the top of the ATA chart, so the Hermetic or mercurial quality of the minister or hierophant is given prominence. The next two signs, Cancer and Leo, and their alchemical metals, silver and gold, represent the goal of unity. Hermes is the third person involved in the process of the *hieros gamos*, or sacred marriage, of king and queen, or Sun and Moon. And it is amazing to recall that in chemical alchemy, the element mercury is the agent that forms an amalgam with silver and gold. This is an extremely vital function, and Mercury/Hermes is a key player. The overall process can be called a Hermetic one, and the astrology and psychology is likewise related to Hermes and his roles of both appreciating duality and re-membering unity, as in putting the two halves back together.

The Hermetic key word that describes Gemini is *synthesizing*. It is Hermes's job and joy to bring the opposites together.

Cancer and the Sixth Chakra

In the ATA of the signs, Cancer and the Moon correspond to the sixth Ajna chakra, esoterically called the third eye. This chakra, also called the guru chakra, is illustrated with two white petals and a central bindu, which can be associated with the two hemispheres of the brain or the two temples of the skull, and the central endocrine glands that produce important hormones. Other names for the hormones produced in this region are "fruits of the Moon tree" and *amrita*, a Sanskrit word that literally means "immortality."

Amrita also refers to nectar and so it is "the nectar of immortality." It is also called ambrosia and soma. Soma is the name of the male Hindu divinity of the Moon, also called Chandra. The crescent Moon is viewed as an arc and the cup or chalice that holds the ambrosia. It is claimed in yoga that, by placing the tongue on the roof of the mouth or palate, one can taste the soma or nectar that results from deep meditation. This understanding from yoga can also be seen as highlighting the importance of the "nectars," or hormones, produced by the pineal and other glands in the head. Solar and lunar light play important roles in the waxing and waning of the production of these hormones, since the third eye, or pineal gland, is sensitive to levels of illumination.

The key Hermetic phrase for Cancer is *compassion.* Like the opalescence of the oyster shell and its pearl, Cancer shines with a lunar glow, like mother-of-pearl, that is the feminine variation on the theme of radiance.

Leo and the Seventh Chakra

In the Alchemical Tantric Arrangement that we have been presenting in this book, Leo corresponds to the highest chakra, located at the top center, or crown, of the human head. It is perhaps no mistake that royal Leo is related to the crown. This is the highest center and corresponds to the most evolved parts of the brain and the subtlest levels of perception. The crown or Sahasrara chakra, at the topmost part of the head, represents the ability to tune in to information beyond the usual borders of physical reality, like auras, subtle bodies, and cosmic intuition. Perhaps the fontanelle, which is an opening in the baby's skull, suggests an opening to the realm from whence the baby came. The word *fontanelle* is etymologically related to the word *fountain,* and one can imagine, during meditation, the energy passing up the spine and out through the top of the head, creating a fountain of light as it shoots out in a golden shower. The glyph for Leo can be seen as representing a snake, which reveals Leo's association with the kundalini serpent energy arisen, culminating as the golden shower.

The roughly spherical human head is like the two celestial orbs of the eclipsed Moon and Sun. Their alchemical marriage, or hieros gamos, is celebrated here in the head's two temples and witnessed by the two eyes plus the third eye. In the image below of the royal marriage between the king and queen of the Greek divinities, Zeus and Hera, we see the alchemical couple accompanied by the Hermetic third person, in this case, appropriately, it is Iris, the eye.

The key phrase of Hermetic Leo is *wisdom.* This sign of the golden

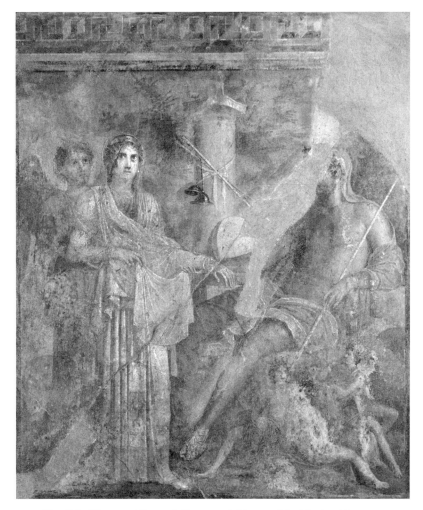

Fig. 5.1. The wedding of Zeus and Hera with Iris looking on.
Fresco in Casa del Poeta Tragico, Pompeii, 1st century CE.

royal crown carries with it the meaning of light and radiance. The Sun brings light, warmth, and life, and spiritually, Leo does the same. As shown above, the symbolism of union, marriage, and oneness is a fundamental meaning of Hermetic Leo.

Virgo and the Fifth Chakra

The powerful pure virginal energy of Virgo is perfect for the first step down in the process of distributing the union or amalgam of Leo and

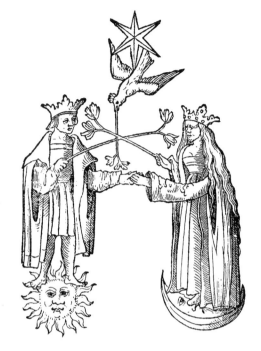

Fig. 5.2. An alchemical
divine marriage, from
Rosarium Philosophorum,
1550.

Cancer's royal gold and silver to the rest of the subtle body, represented by the chakra system. Mercury, in the sign of Gemini, was the minister preparing the way for the alchemical marriage. As ruler of Virgo, Mercury is more attuned to carrying souls on the downward healing path. Seasonally, Virgo comes at the time of harvest, and the divine virgin, like the older feminist myth of earthy Pandora, distributes the gifts of her work in the fields to the people.

The Hermetic key word for Virgo is *distributing,* as in distributing the harvest. The image of Virgo the virgin often portrays her with a plant, sheaf of grain, or ear of corn in her hand.

The fifth chakra, as noted before, is related to the throat and communication center. In this case, in the context of healing, Virgo can be imagined as the communicator of the wholeness represented by the divine marriage of Sol and Luna. It is the profound healing of the golden silence and spaciousness of meditation that communicates the oneness beyond the separate self, which is resonant with the symbolism of the virgin.

Libra and the Fourth Chakra

The qualities of Libra—beauty, balance, harmony, the arts, fairness, and personal relationship—fit well with the fourth, or heart center, chakra. If we imagine that the unified energy of the crown chakra is being distributed downward, in this fourth chakra it falls into the heart, not only as romantic love but also as unconditional love and in its expression as art.

In myth, the ruling planet of Libra, Venus/Aphrodite, goddess of love, has many stories and personas. Two of her names, Urania and Pandemos, describe the qualities of heavenly and conventional love. Aphrodite, together with her husband, Hephaestus, the talented craftsman and metal smith, focus on marriage, relationship, and art. Aphrodite's many other love affairs, and Hephaestus's anguish, paint another kind of picture, one of freedom and passion. It should be noted that Aphrodite is another example of an ancient goddess who does not fare well in patriarchal myth.

The key word of Hermetic Libra is *beautifying*. Art and love both fit into this colorful picture. Although art and intimate relationship can both appear as less than totally harmonious, as the philosopher Hegel expressed it, there is often a struggle from thesis to antithesis to synthesis. It is not always pretty; however, this movement viewed from a larger perspective is perfectly imperfect.

Scorpio and the Third Chakra

The fiery third chakra is located at the navel center and relates to both power and control. Both Scorpio and Aries are signs that fit well with this chakra. Although the fiery warrior god Mars/Ares is powerful enough, Pluto/Hades, divinity of the underworld and the apocalypse, has a more ominous and foreboding persona. With Pluto and Scorpio, there is a connection to death, secrecy, and the dangerous alchemical metal, radioactive plutonium.

The symbolism of the sign Aries on the upward, accumulating path through the signs of the zodiac, accents the aggressive individualistic Mars-related tendencies. With Scorpio, on the downward, distributing side of the zodiacal cycle, the focus is on union and seeing beyond apparent duality. The extremely hot water of Scorpio is like a bath that dissolves away the false distinctions and dualities.

The same is true in terms of Scorpio's sexual connotations. If *sexual* means "to cut" as in the word "section," then in Scorpio the emphasis is on the healing or making whole of sexuality. Is intercourse about two, or one appearing as two? Perhaps we can view one level of sexuality in the story of Hades's abduction of Persephone. In Scorpio, the ultimate outcome is contained in the image of Hades and Persephone as king and queen, co-rulers of the underworld realm. Being forcibly taken by Pluto/Hades to his underworld can feel like those times when we are completely lost: our life is blown apart or our mind is blown by a realization. Being the king and queen of the underworld, on the other hand, suggests that there is a deeper perspective on death available to those who dare to look deeper.

Scorpio energy is often connected with the sexual second chakra; however, Scorpio's form of sexuality has a strong element of third chakra blood-red iron and radioactive plutonium, which conjure images of war, manipulation, control, and sacrifice. Scorpio's sexual sacrifice is dramatized in the story of millions of sperm dying like soldiers in battle or as the unfertilized ovum washed away in the blood of menstruation. Scorpio sexuality is well expressed by the French phrase for orgasm, *le petit mort,* meaning "the little death."

The key word of Hermetic Scorpio is *transformation.* The number 8 of the natural sign of Scorpio, which is also the symbol of infinity, is well described by water's path through rivers, ocean, clouds, rain, and back again. It can be an eddy in the river, a wave on the ocean, a shifting cloud, or a falling raindrop, but nothing is lost or gained. Thus, there is nothing essential that dies; this transformation of the temporary collection of atoms and ideas that the self calls "I" and "me" reveals that thinking of the self as separate is a serious illusion. Scorpio is a portal where we learn to die and especially to die to the fear of death. As the title of Thich Nhat Hanh's book states so directly: *No Death, No Fear.*

Sagittarius and the Second Chakra

Represented by the powerful centaur and ruled by expansive Jupiter, Sagittarius has a strong symbolic resonance with the sexual second chakra, which is located in the area of the genitals and the sacrum. It is a strong energy center and a fitting match for Sagittarius's symbolic animal force of the horse and the power of its gigantic ruling planet, Jupiter. In Greek and Roman myth, Zeus/Jupiter was the progenitor of many children, both with his queen and wife, Hera/Juno, and with many other goddesses and mortals.

Following the healing or, better said, re-membering of wholeness, from the passage through the previous transformative sign, fixed Scorpio, mutable Sagittarius celebrates the meaning of the lofty flaming arrow of exuberant life. Based on the lessons learned through Scorpio regarding death, and especially the letting go of the mistaken notion of being a separate self, life is released like a flaming arrow in Sagittarius. This sign is ruler of the thighs, driving us to more energetic movement. Free of hope and fear, what remains is crazy wisdom.

The key word for Hermetic Sagittarius is *playing*. Every part of Sagittarius is primed for fully playing the game of life: mental-intellectual, physical-athletic, sexual-reproductive, academic-teaching, business-financial—all across the board and field.

Capricorn and the First, or Root, Chakra

In the natural zodiac, Capricorn is found at the highest point, or mid-heaven. However, many Capricorns who have made it to the top of the heap ask themselves: "Is this it? Is this all there is to life . . . wealth, power, and fame?" They then may begin to wonder about another kind of knowledge and the path to wisdom and compassion. In that case, the second half of the image of Capricorn comes into play, with the fish's tail representing submersion into the sea of the unconscious. The element, lead, is related to Saturn, Capricorn's ruling planet, and like the lead sinker of a fishing line, material success can become a heavy weight that pulls them back down to begin another cycle. This second cycle of Capricorn can become the foundation of the symbolic alchemical transmutation of lead into gold.

Referring to the image of the Alchemical Tantric Arrangement, we see that Capricorn, with its metal lead, is now the twelfth sign at the very bottom of the cycle of the zodiac; in fact, the end of this sign is the turning point from revolution on the wheel to entrance onto the path upward toward golden enlightenment. The usual cyclic dualistic path is via the sign Aquarius and following the signs of the zodiac around the wheel. The more direct tantric path of kundalini rising is via Uranus's radioactive metal, uranium. The asteroid, Chiron, with an orbit between Saturn and Uranus, is the key to the portal onto the central path, or sushumna, the direct path. We'll explore the potential of the Chiron portal a bit later.

Capricorn's placement at the bottom of the Alchemical Tantric Arrangement of the signs is fitting with the holidays the sign contains: Christmas, as the birth of the light and Christ consciousness in the darkness of winter's night; New Year's Eve, as the beginning of the new year at midnight in midwinter; and Epiphany, as the time twelve days (read twelve signs and houses) after Christmas when the three wise men (read astrologers) confirm Jesus as the messiah (and probably read his mother, father, and baby Jesus his astrological chart with all the major turning points in his life). Zero degrees of Aries is the natural beginning of the astrological year, but Capricorn cradles the spiritual beginning.

Capricorn, as the twelfth and final sign in the Hermetic order of the zodiac, can be related to the old soul who has seen and experienced so much that she or he is ripe and ready for the direct path. In Tibetan Buddhism, this is called the "old dog" stage, when the old soul, like an old dog, can lie on the ground and let the children play with its ears and tail, as if to say, "whatever."

The key word for Hermetic Capricorn is *completing*. This expresses the cycle or many cycles that Capricorn has experienced and the readiness the sign brings for either beginning a new cycle through the dualistic signs of the zodiac or turning onto the central channel that ultimately points to the heart center and nonduality.

✦

As we go further out in the cosmos, further up the periodic table, further into the center of the tantric chakra system, further down the passage through the gateless gate into the dimensionless central point with no center and no points, representing the void no-thing source of all, what is discovered? This is *it*!

I hope it is clear at this juncture and every juncture that although there appears to be a progression through the signs and through the chakras, ultimately, kundalini has no beginning and no end, so it all points to absolute union of the alpha and the omega.

It should be noted that from the perspective of radical nonduality, what might be called absolute enlightenment means no separation, no self, no duality. Goneness. Never even born!

However, in the dream-like world of Maya, there is apparently cause and effect. Yoga practice can act as a form of hastening evolution, or what might be called awakening kundalini. It is my intuition that, because of the connection of the central axis of the ATA with the story of the serpent kundalini coiled at the base of the root chakra, transits to this cusp between Capricorn and Aquarius can be special times for healing and awakening of latent energy and abilities. In chapter 10 practices are presented that make use of this amazing information.

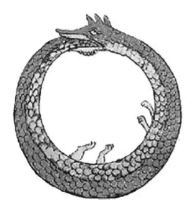

Fig. 5.3. The ouroboros, the snake swallowing its own tail, is a symbol of infinity and wholeness.
Codex Parisinus Graecus, 1478

6

Alchemical and Tantric Chakra Associations

The alchemical arrangement of the signs of the zodiac presented herein highlights their shared rulership, from Saturn and lead at the bottom in the signs of Capricorn and Aquarius to the Moon and silver in Cancer and the Sun and gold in the sign of Leo at the top. This arrangement correlates perfectly with the seven chakras of the tantric system.

There is considerable sexual symbolism involved in the tantric chakra system. The sexual connotations of Tantra are appropriate in the sense of appreciating the totality of human existence, where sexuality is spiritual and the paths up and down the chakras are equally full and empty. Sexual union is a literal and symbolic demonstration of the mystery of oneness and multiplicity, or OM. "Ommmmm" can be interpreted poetically as "O" for Oneness and "mmm" for multiplicity.

As noted in chapter 5, each chakra in the tantric system is represented by a lotus flower. In nature, the flower opens out from the center of the bud and is therefore symbolic of the central point or dimensionless dot that is the unmanifest source, while the blossoming petals are the manifestation—the zero and the many. Each chakra has an axis around which it turns, restating the image of a stationary center and the rotating periphery, the dimensionless dot in the center of the circle, which is a mandala and a symbol for the self, the absolute, no-thing, and everything.

Note that the word *flower,* which is often associated with the yoni (vulva), is also flow-er, again suggesting the yoni as well as birth—the manifest being born or poured out of the unmanifest.

The Buddha is often depicted holding a lotus flower. The tantric chakras accent both the nondual center and the duality of name and form, color and fragrance of the unfolding petals. All of these symbols—the chakras, flowers, the yoni, and mandalas—draw attention to the potent heart center and are ultimately, like the Buddhist heart sutra, about nonduality.

THE ALCHEMY OF THE TRANS-SATURNIAN PLANETS

Medieval alchemists were aware of seven planets in the heavens (including the Sun and Moon) and correlated them with seven metals in the earth. The "accidental" discovery by amateur astronomer William Herschel in 1781 of a new planet opened the way for amazing synchronicity. Johann Bode, a German astronomer who calculated the new planet's orbit, thought that because Saturn had been named after Jupiter's father, the newly discovered planet should be named for Saturn's father, Ouranus, divinity of the heavens. That is how the seventh planet from the Sun got the name Uranus. Uranus is the only planet in our solar system to have been given a Greek name rather than a Roman one. Amazingly, Johann Bode's friend, chemist Martin Klaproth, in support of Bode's name for the new planet, named the new element he discovered around this same time uranium, linking the planet Uranus with the radioactive element uranium. Eventually, astrologers assigned the new and unique planet Uranus as the ruler of the innovative sign Aquarius.

The alignment among the three disciplines of astrology's Rosetta Stone becomes even more striking when the planets beyond Saturn and their radioactive metals are added. When we observe that Uranus relates to the radioactive element, uranium; that the next element in the periodic table, the radioactive element neptunium, correlates with the planet discovered next, Neptune (the new ruler of Pisces); and the radioactive element plutonium, next in the periodic table, correlates with Pluto (the new ruler of Scorpio), then the alignment among the three systems is especially striking.

The amazing progression of the more recently discovered planets and the radioactive elements named for them represents the awakening of kundalini energy. The outer circle of signs of the zodiac and their original ruling planets in the ATA represents the natural cycle of life and its *revolution and evolution;* while the direct inward and upward movement of energy via the Chiron portal and central nadi leads to *involution and evolution.* Although both paths hold potential for the evolution of consciousness, revolution suggests repetition, while involution implies a movement inward to the source, or center.

The symbolic development upward through the chakras is sometimes viewed as a one-way path, going from one to seven. However, the symbolism of the first four chakras and their radioactive alchemical elements also points to a path inward toward the Ultimate Center, represented by the dot in the center of the central heart chakra—a reminder of primordial unity. The dimensionless dot in the center of the heart points toward the unmanifest no-thing that is apparently manifest in the apparent phenomenal world.

THE FIRST FOUR
RADIOACTIVE CHAKRAS

An amazing aspect of the ATA is that the lower four chakras correlate with the outermost planets. These same outer planets were arranged in their natural order for naming radioactive elements in the periodic table of modern chemistry.

Uranus, the first planet beyond Saturn, discovered with the aid of technology, is related to the radioactive metal uranium (element $92 = 9 + 2 = 11$) and is the new planetary ruler of Aquarius, the eleventh sign of the natural zodiac, beginning the upward movement in the tantric arrangement, and is located in the *first, or root, chakra.*

Neptune, beyond Uranus, is the new ruler of the twelfth natural sign, Pisces, and is related to the radioactive metal neptunium (number 93 = 12) in alchemy, located in the *second, or sacral, chakra.*

Pluto, next in the planetary order, is the new dwarf planet ruler of Scorpio and is related to the radioactive metal plutonium (number 94 = 13). Scorpio and Aries are the two signs related to the *third, or navel, chakra* in the ATA.

Eris, the dwarf planet beyond Pluto, can be related to the next radioactive metal in the periodic table, americium (number 95 = 14), and is tentatively located in the fourth, or heart, chakra in the ATA. Eris has strong archetypal resonance to the fourth chakra through her role in the story of the Judgment of Paris.

RADIOACTIVE METALS AND KUNDALINI RISING

The outermost planets, starting with Uranus, the new ruler of the sign Aquarius, are alchemically associated with radioactive metals:

Aquarius, ruled by Uranus, has as its alchemical metal uranium.
Pisces, ruled by Neptune, has the alchemical metal neptunium.
Scorpio, ruled by Pluto, has the alchemical metal plutonium.

I associate these radioactive elements and their related signs and planets with supercharged kundalini energy and the central sushumna nadi.

Uranus, Neptune, and Pluto are therefore associated with the first three chakras. Next in line is the heart chakra, which I have tentatively associated with the new dwarf planet Eris. (I have not yet followed this progression to connect the newly discovered planets out past Eris.) In one sense, the heart is a fitting final goal. However, by continuing up the central path beyond the heart center and its path of love, we come to the three upper chakras, which contain the alchemically symbolic trinity of Mercury/Hermes, the Moon, and the Sun. In alchemical imagery, Mercury/Hermes is the minister who presides over the royal marriage of the lunar queen and solar king, representing the ultimate experience of union, or oneness.

The central sushumna nadi, or direct subtle path, via the highly transformative planets outward from Saturn, correlates with the powerfully transformative radioactive elements. I call this path the direct path to enlightenment, while the cycle around the signs of the zodiac represents the natural path of accumulating awareness and wisdom and then distributing the "gold," or insights, back through repeated cycles. Taken together, the circular path of the signs and the straight path of the central sushumna nadi create the complete spiral of evolution.

THROUGH THE GATELESS GATE AND INTO THE CENTERLESS CENTER

Cycles through the signs and their related chakras are part of the natural evolutionary rebirth cycle. As we follow transits around the wheel of the zodiac and up the straight and narrow central path, we naturally make an evolutionary spiral (horizontal circle of signs plus vertical line of chakras equals spiral of evolution).

However, for those who understand the meaning of a gateless gate, passing through the Chiron portal immediately onto the central kundalini nonpath, consider the following: everything points to the always already existing perfect totality. Meditation is paradoxical in that there is nothing to attain and no separate self to attain it. In Zen, such meditation is called *shikantaza,* roughly meaning "just simply sitting," free of any goals.

7

Chiron as Key
and Bridge

Since I am calling the charged cusp between Capricorn and Aquarius the Chiron portal, it is important to understand more about the qualities of Chiron. The asteroid Chiron orbits between Saturn and Uranus—the crucial point between the ancient, visible planets and the modern planets discovered with the use of telescopes. Chiron was discovered by astronomer Charles Kowal on November 1, 1977. In fact, we know the exact time and location of this discovery, allowing us to create and interpret a chart for Chiron's "birth." We'll examine both a traditional astrology chart for this moment, as well as a Hermetic chart, using the Alchemical Tantric Arrangement to discover even more about Chiron.

Reflecting on the stories in part 1 surrounding the centaur teacher of mythology, it should come as no surprise that Chiron is known by astrologers to emphasize the dual qualities of the wounded healer and the maverick.

The wounded-healer quality can be related to the transit through Capricorn's "dark night of the soul," which offers a basis for understanding the Buddha's emphasis on suffering. Saturn's initiation into the harsh realities of life is like the Buddha's realization of sickness, old age, and death. This, in turn, can allow a person the perspective, with the awakening help of Uranus, to follow his or her own idiosyncratic life path; hence, the other quality of Chiron, the maverick. Chiron's challenges and blessings have to do with uncovering our wounds and traumas so that they might be healed. Such healing allows for freeing up energy to follow our path or dharma and for helping others, which is a good foundation for awakening the spiritual kundalini energy.

Maverick energy is the ability to follow our own inner guidance that comes from uncovering our wounds for healing and having insights into our unconscious conditioning. Such insights, in turn, can result in living up to our full potential and manifesting our greatness, thereby awakening the kundalini energy of spiritual evolution, with its resulting ability to be our true self and ultimately realize no self or union, the true meaning of yoga.

Kristine J. Anselmo and Monte J. Zerger's article "Chiron: Full Spectrum," published in the *Mountain Astrologer,* focuses on the phrase *key and bridge.* Their discovery chart of Chiron accents it as the singleton in the bucket or funnel pattern, pointing to this centaur planetoid as a point of focus for all the other planets.

Another meaning of Chiron as key and bridge is shown through the Alchemical Tantric Arrangement. Chiron is the *key* to unlocking the central nadi in the chakra system and a *bridge* between the downward and upward paths of the zodiac signs. (See figure 7.1.)

TRADITIONAL CHART INTERPRETATION OF CHIRON'S DISCOVERY

An examination of the chart for the moment of Chiron's discovery can reveal much about this asteroid's nature. For more information on interpreting charts, look to part 3 of this book. The following interpretations are a good example to familiarize yourself with the new dimensions offered by the application of the ATA.

In this case, the discovery chart of Chiron contains an obvious opposition between Chiron and the Sun, which is shining the light of

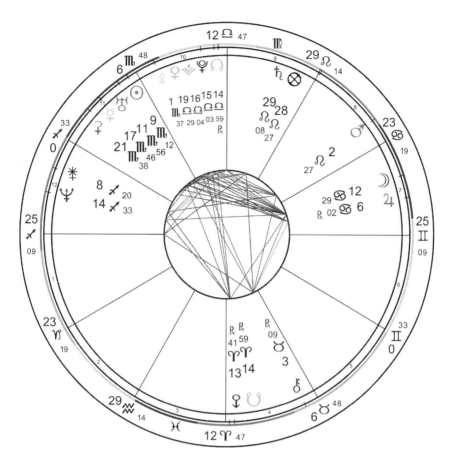

Fig. 7.1. Chiron discovery chart of November 1, 1977, 9:56 a.m.,
in Pasadena, California, by astronomer Charles Kowal

discovery directly on Chiron. Additionally, there is a square to Mars in an obvious fixed T-square. The two outer, highly transformative planets, Pluto conjunct Rahu in Libra and Eris conjunct Ketu in Aries, square to the Moon and Jupiter in Cancer, complete this dramatic formation. Note the placement of Eris accented in the foundational fourth house alongside Chiron, suggesting a special connection between these two. Note also the positive aspects to Chiron and the cardinal T-square with Eris opposite Pluto, conjunct the nodes, and square to rulers Moon and Jupiter conjunct.

HERMETIC CHART INTERPRETATION
OF CHIRON'S DISCOVERY

The Hermetic astrology chart is not meant to replace the standard astrology chart. However, it is a revealing addition to the overall astrological interpretation.

Notice, in the Hermetic chart how the basic T-square emphasizes the important planets in the sixth and seventh chakras: Jupiter and the Moon, both energized in Cancer, and Mars and Saturn in Leo. My Hermetic interpretation would certainly include how the newly discovered planetoid Chiron has an important alchemical and tantric role to play. This is accented by the alchemical emphasis on the lunar queen

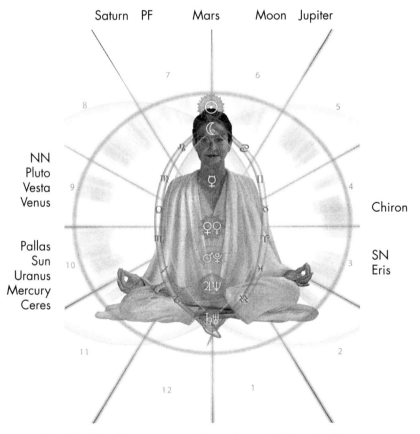

Fig. 7.2. The Hermetic astrology chart of Chiron's discovery,
November 1, 1977

in Cancer meeting the strong masculine energy of Mars and Saturn in royal Leo at the crown chakra. The Hermetic chart thereby suggests a goal of transforming the energy of Mars and Saturn to their highest vibration, ultimately as warriors for enlightenment.

Chiron the asteroid—named for the wise centaur, universal teacher and healer, and symbolizing the union of the powerful elegant horse and the human warrior—is appropriately placed in the lovely fourth, or heart, chakra of this chart. This fourth chakra is related to the upward path of healing love and is also the final goal of unconditional love because it is centrally located in the chakra system. The many planets in Libra also accent the fourth, or heart, chakra. Libra puts emphasis on truth, beauty, art, and relationship, all qualities contributing to Chiron's healing abilities.

Strong activation of the third, or navel, chakra in the Hermetic chart is in tune with Chiron's animal power. Involving plenty of Scorpio, it suggests that Chiron's healing power has a strong sexual connotation and also a penetration into other mysteries such as death and radical transformation. Let us recall that Chiron was also said to be a great astrologer. In Chiron's Hermetic chart, Eris in Aries adds to third chakra intensity, as a warrior for justice, especially with the south node nearby.

THE CHIRON PORTAL

In Alchemical Tantric Astrology, while the cycle of the zodiac can be related to the ida and pingala nadis, as we noted before, Chiron can be seen as activating the portal on the cusp of Capricorn and Aquarius at the root center, opening to the central sushumna kundalini nadi. Thus, although it can be helpful to track all the planets and asteroids as they transit through the signs and chakras, the planets Saturn and Uranus and the asteroid Chiron take on special meaning as guardians of the threshold, since they are found at the gateway to the central kundalini channel. They represent symbolically the transition from inert lead, the container, to radioactive uranium, the initiator of the Atomic Age, at the charged cusp between the signs Capricorn and Aquarius at the bottom of the ATA. Chiron, represented by the wise centaur archer and healer, being both animal and human, is a fitting image for this bridging transition between the two quite different signs, Capricorn and Aquarius; two quite different planets, Saturn and Uranus; and the downward and upward paths of the two channels, pingala and ida.

Because Saturn, Chiron, and Uranus are related to the gateway between the invisible and visible planets, the three nadis, or tantric channels, and the beginning of the radioactive elements, their transits take on special relevance. (See Barbara Hand Clow's *Astrology and the Rising of Kundalini: The Transformative Power of Saturn, Chiron, and Uranus.*) The Moon's nodes, Rahu and Ketu, are also especially relevant.

The roughly three cycles of Saturn's 28 to 30 years in an average human life, Chiron's two 50-year cycles, Uranus's four cycles of 21 years, and four or five of the nodes's roughly 18.5-year cycles take on extra meaning because they suggest charged initiatory times in the tantric evolutionary, involutionary process. These four, Saturn, Chiron, Uranus, and the Moon's nodes, are the heavy hitters at the very beginning of the alchemical, tantric progression.

In 2020, the alignment of the two solar system giants, Jupiter and Saturn, exactly on the Chiron portal portended a dramatically propitious moment regarding an opening of the Chiron, or kundalini, portal. We were expecting some especially intense times around 2020, which have indeed been both extremely challenging and spiritually enriching; however, the worldwide events around this time have been absolutely mind-boggling.

8

The Hermetic Houses

Alchemical Tantric Astrology, by the simple but profound "turn of the dial," created a unique new astrological system. Although astrology has always had a focus on spiritual development, this new system of astrology reveals a non-arbitrary form of yoga represented by the seven chakras. The twelve houses of traditional astrology have a definite story to tell in their progression, and the newly revealed houses of the ATA offer an even more effective path to wisdom and ultimate union.

HERMETIC ASTROLOGY NUMBERING

Numbers are a vital and an essential part of transiting numerically through the twelve signs of the zodiac. Numbers have a depth of meaning that puts them in Hermes's realm because as the messenger of the divinities, he is both the interpreter and the keeper of secret messages. His herald's staff, the caduceus, is similar to the image of the tantric chakras of the subtle body, and its form has a symbolic message of esoteric knowledge, democratic values, and healing.

Each number, with its associated sacred geometry, carries profound messages. We are looking here at the numerical messages of the twelve signs as they are arranged according to their alchemical and tantric order. Hermetic numbering begins with Aquarius, the first sign of the ascending, accumulating side of the zodiac and is associated with the first, or root, chakra and ends with Capricorn, the twelfth and final sign of the ATA.

Although the number of the sign and house based on the natural order of the zodiac (Aries as the first sign and first natural house and Pisces as the twelfth sign and the twelfth natural house) is still relevant, the Hermetic order of the Alchemical Tantric Arrangement adds other spiritual dimensions of meaning to the signs and houses.

The first house of all Hermetic astrology charts begins appropriately at the bottom, in the root chakra, in the sign of Aquarius, which is therefore the first sign and house of the ATA system. Hermetic astrology is therefore Aquarian in nature, making Saturn and Uranus, the ruling planets of Aquarius, the overall rulers of this and every Hermetic astrology chart. Saturn, whose alchemical metal is lead, is like the container, while the alchemical metal of Uranus, uranium, is the highly reactive radioactive agent of transformation. Thus, the Hermetic chart highlights the potential for the evolution of human consciousness after many cycles of experience (Capricorn) and a radical awakening shift (Aquarius). When an individual's natal data is appropriately entered, the Hermetic chart can be read for the planetary relations to the various chakras, offering pointers for the timing of individual evolution.

There is another suggestive piece of the puzzle found in the fact that if we were to think of the tenth Hermetic house, which is occupied by the sign Scorpio, as the *natural* first house of the chart, then Scorpio would be the rising sign and Pluto would be the ruler of the chart. In a sense therefore the Hermetic chart is both an Aquarian and a Scorpionic chart!

THE PATH OF THE HERMETIC CYCLE

The Hermetic cycle can be seen as six ascending, accumulating signs from Aquarius to Cancer and six descending, distributing signs from Leo to Capricorn (6 + 6 = 12). We can also consider the Hermetic cycle as seven ascending, accumulating signs from Aquarius to Leo. The signs Cancer and Leo, with their ruling planets Moon and Sun and alchemical metals silver and gold, have a propensity for joining together in an alchemical union or marriage. Called electrum, this new combination of their alchemical metals is then symbolically distributed down through the remaining five signs and five elements, ether, air, fire, water, and earth, from Virgo to Capricorn (7 + 5 = 12). It should be noted that the division of 12 into 7 and 5 is common, as in the twelve signs, seven chakras, seven traditional planets, and five elements.

This cycle of either six or seven signs is simplified to more easily demonstrate the relationships among the signs of the zodiac and the seven chakras. However, in the *Ashtanga Yoga Primer* by Baba Hari Dass, a more detailed interwoven description is given. A spiraling around the chakras is suggested by the alternation of masculine signs (fire and air) and feminine signs (earth and water), as we move around the zodiac and up and down the two channels represented by the two serpents.

The following is a brief journey through the twelve numbers of the Hermetic zodiac:

1. **Aquarius: First Hermetic house. Number One, the first.** First, or root, chakra. New ruler, Uranus; alchemical metal, uranium. Traditional ruler, Saturn; alchemical metal, lead. Aquarius ushers in the springtime opening of the cycle. Key word, *awakening.*

2. **Pisces: Second Hermetic house. Number Two, duality.** Second, or sacral, chakra. New ruler, Neptune; alchemical metal, neptunium. Traditional ruler, Jupiter; alchemical metal, tin. Pisces is known for watery emotional merging. Key word, *fertilizing.*

3. **Aries: Third Hermetic house. Number Three, trinity.** Third, or navel, chakra. New ruler, Pluto; alchemical metal, plutonium. Traditional ruler, Mars; alchemical metal, iron. Aries is associated with fiery activity. Key word, *activating.*

4. **Vacca/Taurus: Fourth Hermetic house. Number Four, quaternity.** Fourth, or heart, chakra. New ruler, Eris; alchemical metal, americium. Traditional ruler, Venus; alchemical metal, copper. Loving relationships and sensuality are accented. Key word, *nurturing.*

5. **Gemini: Fifth Hermetic house. Number Five, quintessence.** Fifth, or throat, chakra. Ruler, Mercury; alchemical metal, mercury. The hierophant. Communication accented. Key word, *synthesizing.*

6. **Cancer: Sixth Hermetic house. Number Six, family.** Sixth, brow,

or Ajna, chakra. Ruler, the Moon; alchemical metal, silver. Lunar queen and mother-of-pearl. Key word, *compassion*.

7. **Leo: Seventh Hermetic house. Number Seven, fortune.** Seventh, or crown, chakra. Ruler, the Sun; alchemical metal, gold. Wise king. Key word, *wisdom*.

8. **Virgo: Eighth Hermetic house. Number Eight, infinity.** Fifth, or throat, chakra. Ruler, Mercury; alchemical metal, mercury. Harvest goddess. Notice that the "harvest" distributed by the Virgo goddess is now symbolically the alchemical electrum of the divine marriage (hieros gamos) of the solar king and lunar queen; the sixth and seventh chakras are now united, and the downward path continues from the throat chakra. Key word, *distributing*.

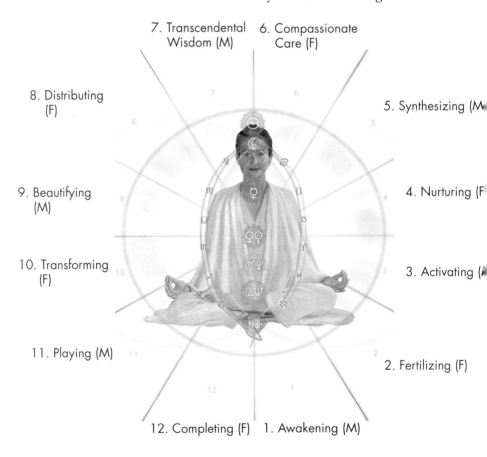

Fig. 8.1. Hermetic numbering

9. **Libra: Ninth Hermetic house. Number Nine, harmony.** Fourth, or heart, chakra. Ruler, Venus; alchemical metal, copper. Art is utilized to share the insights of the divine marriage. Harmony, beauty, unconditional love. Key word, *beautifying*.

10. **Scorpio: Tenth Hermetic house. Number Ten, wholeness.** Third, or navel, chakra. Ruler, Pluto; alchemical metal, plutonium. Key word, *transforming*.

11. **Sagittarius: Eleventh Hermetic house. Number Eleven, mastery.** Second, or sacral, chakra. Ruler, Jupiter; alchemical metal, tin. Intelligence, play, leela, enjoyment. Key word, *playing*.

12. **Capricorn: Twelfth Hermetic house. Number Twelve, totality.** First, or root, chakra. Ruler, Saturn; alchemical metal, lead. Final matters, completion, wisdom of experience. Key word, *completing*.

Notice in figure 8.1 that each chakra has a masculine air and fire sign and a feminine water and earth sign associated, designated by M and F. The movement up and down the chakras therefore describes two spirals, similar to the twin serpents on Hermes's staff.

9

Tracking
the Cosmic Serpent

The Caduceus, Eclipses, DNA, and Siddhis

Contemplating the various threads of knowledge contained in this book for more than forty years, various insights have become apparent. Perhaps the most exciting has come from the profound symbolism of the cosmic serpent. I wanted to understand how astrology, alchemy, and yoga functioned together, which kept wrapping me in the coils of a giant snake or dragon . . . by which I mean that the symbolism of the serpent kept appearing and in turn led me to the serpentine DNA double helix and beyond.

THE SERPENT PATHS OF THE ALCHEMICAL TANTRIC ARRANGEMENT

In figure 9.1, progression through the signs of the zodiac is represented by a silver serpent and a gold serpent moving in opposite directions. The ascending, accumulating path from Aquarius through Cancer, shown on the left, classically feminine side of the human body, is associated with the lunar ida nadi, and the descending, distributing path from Leo back down the right side of the human body to Capricorn is associated with the solar pingala nadi. These two complementary paths around the zodiac correlate with the circulation of prana, or life energy, during our natural life process, similar to the inhalation and exhalation of the breath. It is noteworthy that *prana,* like the Chinese *chi,* can be translated as "electricity."

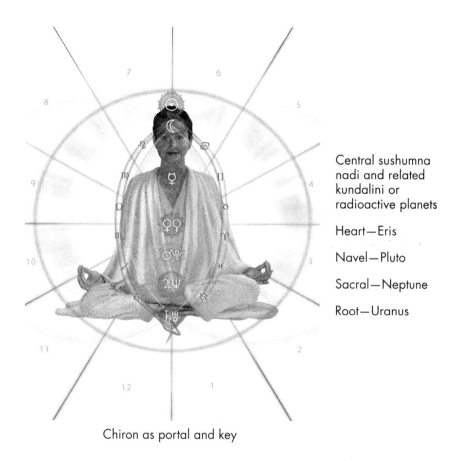

Central sushumna nadi and related kundalini or radioactive planets

Heart—Eris

Navel—Pluto

Sacral—Neptune

Root—Uranus

Chiron as portal and key

Fig. 9.1. Three paths: the two serpents containing the zodiac signs and a central path of chakras with associated planets

In ashtanga yoga, the classical eight-limbed yoga, one limb is called pranayama, or breath control. In this practice, it is said that when the ida and pingala nadis are balanced, then the central sushumna nadi is more active. The ashtanga yoga pranayama called *nadishodhana,* or alternate nostril breathing, is practiced to facilitate this balance.

The third path, via the sushumna nadi, is associated with the central axis of the Hermetic astrology chart. I associate the asteroid Chiron with the beginning of this central channel in the root chakra. This association came from the understanding that Chiron's cycle of fifty years falls between Saturn's twenty-eight to thirty-year cycle and Uranus's eighty-four-year cycle, Saturn and Uranus being the ruling planets of Capricorn and Aquarius. Chiron, therefore, forms a bridge between the visible planets, of which Saturn is the last, and the outer transcendental planets, which begin with Uranus. Saturn and Uranus are the two ruling planets of the root, or first, chakra.

Another serpent within the Hermetic chart is the dragon, represented by the lunar nodes. These nodes are known as the head and tail of the dragon, or Rahu and Ketu in Vedic astrology, and are strongly associated with the root chakra and the kundalini serpent. As we saw in figure 7.1, the nodes were accented at the time of Chiron's discovery, appropriately located at the top and bottom, or crown and root, of the chart and conjunct the potent opposition between Pluto and Eris. As will be shown when we explore some chart interpretations below, this opposing pair of lunar nodes, which relate to eclipse events, have an important role to play in the ATA. And once again, they are symbolically resonant with the Cosmic Serpent and with kundalini because they are the head and tail of a serpent or dragon.

THE CADUCEUS AND THE HERMETIC CHART

The caduceus, or Hermes's herald staff, is commonly depicted in the form of two serpents wrapped around a central rod, similar to the tantric yoga subtle body created through meditations such as in chapter 10. Hermes's staff and the usual image of the yoga chakras show the two outer channels spiraling around the central rod. This spiral is especially important because of its resonance with the DNA double helix (figure 9.4).

The straight silver and gold snakes of the Hermetic astrology chart are used only to make the relationship to the signs of the zodiac easier to demonstrate. Many occult researchers have noted similarities among the images of the subtle body in tantric yoga, the staff or caduceus of Hermes/Mercury, and the double helix of the DNA molecule. All three of these powerfully transformative images include serpent symbolism, and thereby offer profound hints about their connections.

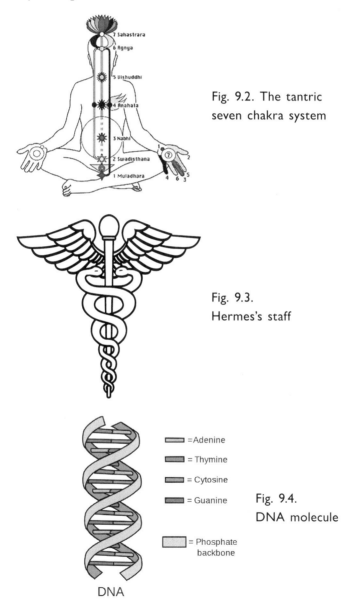

Fig. 9.2. The tantric seven chakra system

Fig. 9.3. Hermes's staff

= Adenine
= Thymine
= Cytosine
= Guanine   Fig. 9.4.
DNA molecule
= Phosphate backbone

DNA

DNA AND THE CHAKRAS

The Alchemical Tantric Arrangement of the signs of the zodiac accents a central axis between Capricorn and Aquarius at the base of the astrological wheel and between Cancer and Leo at the top. This allows us to discover a progression of seven ruling planets from Saturn to the Sun and thence to associate the seven alchemical metals from lead to gold and finally the seven chakras of tantric yoga. With the introduction of yoga in the larger sense of the eightfold path of ashtanga yoga, expanded realms of psychological and spiritual development are revealed. One suggestive example of this revealing multidimensional connection involves the serpent theme, which incorporates the Cosmic Serpent of mythology and anthropology, the kundalini serpent of tantric yoga, and the DNA molecular "serpent."

The seven traditional planets, alchemical metals, and chakras represent a developmental path from highly conditioned behavior to wisdom and freedom. Tantric, or kundalini, yoga adds another dimension, symbolized by the planets outward from Saturn and their associated radioactive alchemical metals, uranium, neptunium, and plutonium. The tantric symbolism of kundalini as a serpent, illustrated coiled around a phallic lingam in the area at the base of the spine, is a rich suggestive image and has been associated with the serpentine double helix of the DNA crystal, as we will see below.

The book by Jeremy Narby, *The Cosmic Serpent: DNA and the Origins of Knowledge,* is helpful for navigating this next step of the journey by bringing together correspondences between the art and descriptions of Cosmic Serpents by Amazonian shamans and DNA genetic science.

To summarize the most relevant parts of this fascinating book: Narby ingested ayahuasca with a shaman in the Amazon and during a terrifying experience saw brightly colored serpents in his visions. He also learned from the shaman that during such visionary experiences, shamans are sometimes taught the qualities of healing or poisoning from the plants themselves. As an anthropologist, Narby was highly intrigued by how plants might be able to communicate with humans, which led him to a further study of anthropological records. He read of Amazonian shamans saying that in the human brain, between the two hemispheres, there are twin serpents, and in the beginning of their culture, their ancestors arrived in boats shaped like huge serpents. Narby started to wonder, "Could the twin snakes be referring to the twin strands of the DNA? After all, wasn't the DNA molecule the same for every living species on earth, all coded with the same four compounds designated by the letters A, G, C, and T? Perhaps plants could communicate from their DNA to human DNA."

Turning to mythology, Narby found that the Aztecs said that in the beginning there was a serpent that gave birth to twins, one being Quetzalcoatl, translated as meaning either "feathered serpent" or "magnificent twin." He found myths from around the world with the primal creator being a serpent, such as the rainbow snake of the Australian Aborigines.

Following the hint that shamans around the world communicate with spirits via music and sound that translate into images and finding the book *Ayahuasca Visions* by Luna and Amaringo, he and his friends in the sciences were shocked at what they now saw—beautiful art with images that reminded them of genetic biology.

Next came the science lesson. Reading Francis Crick, co-discoverer of the structure of DNA, Narby learned that Crick believed the DNA molecule to be way too complex to have evolved on Earth, but rather like an extraterrestrial, DNA may have come from the greater cosmos. Hence, not unlike the shamans of the Amazon, Crick envisioned the twin strands of the molecule of life flying onto Earth like a winged double serpent!

Following this, Narby discovered that the DNA molecule when straightened out was about two yards long and only ten atoms wide and was coiled (like kundalini) to fit inside the nucleus of a cell, in volume, about two-millionths of a pinhead. DNA from all the cells in a human being, laid end to end, would stretch to about 125 billion miles. The Cosmic Serpent has been referred to mythically as the axis mundi, or axis of the world, a fitting title for a filament that would wrap around the Earth five million times. Transcription enzymes that read the DNA text to create vital proteins only read the sections called genes, which make up only about 3 percent of the total genome, the function of the other 97 percent is largely unknown—leaving much to the imagination!

Narby also found that the DNA molecule is a crystal that transports electrons efficiently and emits photons or light in the visual spectrum, suggesting a form of knowledge transmission, which has been studied by scientists who note that although the light emitted is weak, it is coherent like lasers.

So, following the trail of the Cosmic Serpent from world myth to Hermes's caduceus, through the jungles with Amazonian shamans to the modern science of genetics, we find ourselves in hot pursuit of the "sacred thread" (reminiscent of Ariadne's thread) that unites all these seemingly disparate realms. In answer to the question of how the Amazonian shamans could learn directly from the plants and what the other 97 percent of the DNA molecule might be about, there comes this amazing suggestion from ancient India . . .

DNA AND YOGIC POWERS

Several thousands of years ago in India, it was already known that via practices of yoga, certain powers or siddhis could be expected. Patanjali is credited with writing down the primary information of yoga in the form of the yoga sutras about 400 CE in four chapters or books called *padas*. The third chapter, or pada, titled "Vibuti Pada," with fifty-six sutras, is focused on the yogic powers, or siddhis, the yogi can expect to appear and contains a warning not to use the powers because they can lead the serious aspirant away from the final goal of yoga, which is total union.

The first *vibuti sutra* (pada 3, sutra 16) states that the yogi can attain the power, or siddhi, of the knowledge of past, present, and future by intense focus, or *samyana,* on the nature of change. The second sutra (pada 3, sutra 17) states that the yogi can learn the meaning of every sound made by all beings by samyana on sound. This could refer to the kind of powers that the shamans of the Amazon develop via various intense shamanic practices to learn directly from plants and animals.

Although we are warned not to take advantage of these siddhis (there are about twenty-one listed in the yoga sutras), these amazing powers are very seductive, to say the least. How many yoga students have fantasized about having some of the storied abilities of great yogis? Knowledge of these siddhis has led me to review several unique experiences in my own life when highly unusual or even miraculous events occurred. Of particular interest in terms of this book, was the time around my thirtieth birthday, on the Spanish island of Formentera, which is mentioned briefly above and described in detail in chapter 12. Many years ago when I was first pondering the questions that led to writing this book, the following query presented itself: "What might have occurred to create this unusual experience?" Below are some of the questions and answers that appeared . . .

What if the DNA crystal, like many other crystals, has the ability to hold information, and what if this crystal, from its travels throughout the cosmos, could be fantastically knowledgeable, might we even say super wise? What if the 97 percent of the DNA molecule, not presently understood as to its purpose, contains information about how to turn on miraculous powers? What if the DNA molecule, or more precisely, the 125 billion miles of DNA in a human body, has a type of intelligence allowing it to assess an intense situation and deem it worthy of activating the extra abilities required to survive or excel?

Although some of the more amazing experiences in my life might be related to ingestion of powerful plants or chemicals, my time on the island of Formentera did not involve any drug experiences, unless eating crushed nettles counts. (I had read that the Tibetan yoga master Milarepa stayed alive by eating nettles. I found that I could crush them in a paper bag to prevent getting stung.) Rather than a drug experience, in this case, it is important to take a closer look at some of the events that occurred leading up to my "hearing the heavenly choirs." It was indeed quite an amazing time for many reasons. I have deeply pondered this time period, and I believe it gives insight into the kinds of events that are related to acquiring powers or siddhis. The following is a list of the events in my life I contemplated in this way:

Studying meditation with Zen teacher Suzuki Roshi in California

My time in the U.S. Navy, which included a year in Vietnam going up and down the rivers of the Mekong Delta, definitely a year of high stress.

Traveling back from Vietnam alone and visiting various sacred sites in S.E. Asia and meditation in Japan. Returning to Hawaii and camping alone on a deserted beach.

Returning to UCSC to complete my B.A. in psychology, I helped build a large redwood labyrinth, an alchemical project.

This project led to meeting Himalayan Yogi Baba Hari Dass and beginning a dedicated study of ashtanga yoga, which involved many challenging practices.

Traveling across the United States en route to Europe, where I visited sacred sites while hitchhiking, and camping.

Dealing with the death of my mother and several other close relatives during this period.

Separation from a longtime sexual partner and beginning my longest period of voluntary celibacy.

Living alone in a small cottage on the island of Formentera for several months, where I had plenty of quiet time for reading spiritual books, doing hatha yoga, fasting, and meditating on "inner sounds."

It became clear that the period of time leading up to and including my experience on Formentera contained elements that were intense and unusual enough to signal the turning on of some extra abilities. I gleaned further insights into the meaning and possible cause of such extraordinary abilities by reading Dean Radin's book *Supernormal: Science, Yoga, and the Evidence for Extraordinary Psychic Abilities.* I understood more about these abilities by reading Baba Hari Dass's, autobiography, *Path Unfolds*, which reveals an amazing range of extraordinary people with extraordinary abilities, who Babaji met in his life in India.

I feel very blessed to have had my extraordinary experience on Formentera and am especially glad about where it has led me. It is also clear that it was not a step toward ultimate enlightenment, unfortunately! When I shared my story with Baba Hari Dass, he did not seem impressed and affirmed that extraordinary experiences and powers are not necessary for yoga, nor is extreme asceticism.

Whether or not it turns out that my intuition is correct regarding the connection of siddhis lying dormant inside our DNA, it is clear that the symbolism of the Cosmic Serpent is somehow symbolically involved, as are intense experiences. Looking closely at the ashtanga yoga practice I learned from Baba Hari Dass, several aspects of this practice fall into this category of "intense." I started with purification exercises, practicing various forms of physical cleansing beside the usual, including vomiting, purging, enemas, swallowing a long cloth, putting a string in my nose that came out my mouth, pouring water in my nostrils, and staring at a candle flame without blinking.

Some of the most accessible ways to create intense experiences involve various forms of fasting, such as holding the breath and not eating, drinking, or sleeping for extended periods. Yogic breathing exercises, or pranayama, include forms of holding and controlling the breath. Various ceremonies I attended involved extended periods of chanting, visualizations, and meditation, including all-night and extended periods of not sleeping and not moving. Fasting from food is a common practice. Following Baba Hari Dass's example of not speaking, I went several months without speaking and only writing on a small slate. (I found it very difficult to argue with my girlfriend as I was limited to just pushing extra hard on the chalk. Ha!)

Both traveling and isolation can provide an ordeal by which new states can be accessed. In my case, I did extensive hitchhiking, which can be very stressful, especially in inclement weather and when stuck in one place for a long time without a ride. I lived alone and traveled alone. It is a form of yoga practice to go on extended pilgrimages. I once heard Baba Hari Dass tell a person to continue his pilgrimage for another year. And, of course, there is the intense experience of taking mind-altering plants, drugs, and drinks when it comes to activating siddhis.

Psychoactive mushrooms and cacti come to mind since they are close to being deadly poisonous and are therefore likely to cause very fearful reactions in the body. A particularly instructive example is the taking of ayahuasca, the South American brew, often led by a native shaman. It includes many of the intense practices mentioned above, possibly including a strange and potentially dangerous jungle setting, exotic customs and languages, a drink made from jungle plants that can produce vomiting and purging, and the possibility of having visions of giant snakes and other strange jungle beings. As mentioned by Jeremy Narby in his book *The Cosmic Serpent,* there are many aspects of the ayahuasca experience relating it to the DNA double helix including seeing visions of images that scientists later identified in art work as resembling genetic material. One striking aspect of the experience is that it involves the utilization of the twisted jungle vine, *Banisteriopsis caapi,* source of one of the active ingredients in the psychoactive brew. (A banister is the handrail at the side of a staircase, and I might add, it could be a spiral staircase! Note the suggestive shape of the vine. There is also the amazing synchronicity of the botanist after whom the vine is named having the last name of Banister!)

The fascinating subject of siddhis or powers could provide enough material for another book or several books; however, in this context, I am following the hints contained in the amazing Christmas comet eclipse event of 1973, hints both in the astrology of multiple rare events that happened in the time of Capricorn 1973 and my unusual experience of hearing "the music of the spheres." It is as if I were following the trail (or is it the tail?) of the serpent kundalini through all the stories of the mythic Cosmic Serpent as it slithered toward the DNA molecule, and finally to the siddhis of the yoga sutras. So, what exactly is it about yoga practice that makes it more likely that some of these siddhis may appear? Apparently, it involves extremely intense and challenging experiences in conjunction with a belief system that supports a positive outcome rather than a negative medical or psychiatric outcome.

10

AstroYoga

The Chakras as
Multidimensional Portals

As I pointed out above, each lotus-shaped chakra functions as a mandala, which is a word borrowed from India to suggest a geometric form that supports contemplation and meditation. In the yoga community I would help with creating multicolored *yantras,* or geometric sand paintings, for meditative use with yoga ceremonies. There are many surprising lessons you can discover as you engage in a meditation practice, especially combined with visualizations.

One lesson that I have learned is that there really are no free lunches, so anything that you do in the spirit of getting or attaining something will need to be paid for down the line. Ha!

The following visualizations have two subtle lessons: The first is based on the alchemical maxim "as above, so below." Just as the cycle of precession can take 26,000 years and Pluto's cycle takes 250 years, each breath can also be a complete cycle as we visualize inhaling up through six signs, then holding the breath as the Moon and Sun are joined in the divine marriage, and then the breath is visualized as returning down the other six signs back to the root chakra.

The second lesson puts the emphasis on union, or oneness. There are three parts of the cycle of visualizations with this emphasis on union:

1. the tantric lingam and yoni/lotus at the base of the spine;
2. the aforementioned alchemical union of Moon and Sun, silver and gold, in the highest chakras; and
3. the final union of breath and nonduality in the center of the heart chakra.

Much in the following contemplations came from my experiences with Baba Hari Dass and his teachings. My personal contributions have come from seeing how yoga can be combined with astrology to create something that benefits from their synergy. From this, I have developed AstroYoga, a yogic meditation practice based on the discoveries of the Alchemical Tantric Arrangement. Those who know yoga and other ceremonial traditions will see that I have borrowed from several traditions in addition to having some ideas come by way of personal intuition. In an American fashion, I invite you to draw on your own sources of creativity and intuition in the following.

ASTROYOGA
INTEGRATED MEDITATION

A person can attune to the alchemical tantric process as represented in figure 10.1 with little knowledge of AstroYoga. Conversely, if the individual is quite knowledgeable by being aware of the planets in her or his Hermetic chart, then via transits and progressions through the various signs and their related chakras, she or he can utilize the subtle assistance of each planet's energies. One can benefit from these meditations whether one is a beginner or advanced yoga practitioner.

This meditation can be done at any time by anyone. However, depending on each person's astrology and the transits of his or her own chart, certain times may be especially appropriate, such as when there are transits over the central axis and channel between Capricorn-Aquarius and Cancer-Leo. The planets and other celestial presences most relevant to the Alchemical Tantric Arrangement are particularly

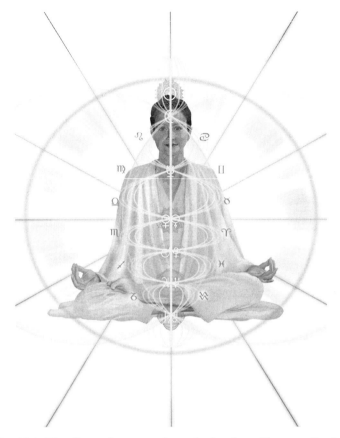

Fig. 10.1. The flow of energy through the AstroYoga meditation

potent in this way: Saturn, Chiron, Uranus, the Sun, the Moon, and the nodes of the Moon.

The following suggestions should be taken as hints only; the basic idea is to utilize various modes in an integrated and synergetic way. For example, the hatha yoga asanas can be used to emphasize the part of the body related to each of the chakras in order. The seed mantra of each chakra can be used, as well as the signs of the zodiac, planets, stars, and constellations.

Four basic forms of visualization are listed below:

1. Circulate energy around the outside of the subtle body through the twelve signs.

2. Bring the energy up the central channel and out the top of the head, then let it shower and spiral down the outside of the subtle body.
3. Bring the energy up through the seven chakras in order, from root to crown.
4. Bring the energy into the central dot, or bindu, of the heart chakra, focusing on the breath.

The first basic form of visualization listed above involves four purifications (1A, 1B, 1C, 1D), inspired by the *Ashtanga Yoga Primer* by my teacher Baba Hari Dass and enhanced by images from the ATA.

✸ 1A. Circulating the Energy

This visualization is based on combining the pranayama, or breathing exercise, of alternate nostril breathing while following the circle of zodiac signs in the ATA. Begin by focusing on the ida nadi, related to the left side of the human body. Hold your right nostril closed with your right thumb and visualize the ascending signs—Aquarius, Pisces, Aries, Vacca/Taurus, Gemini, Cancer, and Leo.

Say the mantra *hang-sa* (meaning, "I am that") silently or count the numbers I through 7 silently while inhaling through the left nostril. Upon reaching the sixth and seventh chakras and the alchemical marriage of the Moon and the Sun, retain the breath and hold closed both nostrils for a count of seven.

Release only your right thumb, keeping the left nostril closed. Exhale through the right nostril: carry an experience of the union of Sun and Moon back down the right side of your subtle body via the pingala nadi. Silently say the mantra *so-hang* ("That I am") or silently count the numbers I through 7 as you descend through the signs: Leo, Virgo, Libra, Scorpio, Sagittarius, and Capricorn.

Repeat this process in the opposite direction. Inhale through the right nostril from Capricorn up to the union of Leo and Cancer, hold the breath, and then exhale out the left nostril while you visualize the energy moving from the union of Leo and Cancer back down from Gemini to Aquarius. This exercise may be repeated three times or as many times as you wish. This exercise is helpful for balancing the energy in the two nadis, ida and pingala.

❋ *1B. Skull Shining*

The second purification exercise, emphasizes the brow, or Ajna, chakra. First, inhale, and follow with quick forced exhalations. In this way, exchange a series of breaths, with the emphasis on exhalation and allowing the inhalation to follow naturally.

Focus on the brow/third eye; visualize air tapping behind the third eye, while silently repeating the mantra *thang*, imitating the sound of a bell ringing inside the skull.

Do this process as long as you wish.

❋ *1C. Fire Wash*

The third purification exercise focuses on the third, or fire, chakra in the area of the navel. Exhale completely and pull the stomach up and in as many times as is comfortable with the breath held out. With each stomach lift repeat the mantra *rang* silently, and visualize fiery energy being circulated throughout the body.

❋ *1D. Horse Mudra*

The fourth purification exercise brings the energy down to the root chakra. Hold the inhalation while tightening and releasing the anal sphincter as many times as is comfortable. Say the mantra *lang* silently.

The following three steps provide visualizations for guiding and concentrating the energy.

❋ *Second Movement—Golden Fountain*

After bringing the wonderful energy of the alchemical marriage of the Sun and Moon down again to the root chakra, visualize the energy of union moving from there back up the central sushumna nadi in the center of the spine as a golden light.

The energy flows upward and out the top of the crown chakra showering like a fountain of light as it descends all around the subtle body as two intertwining serpents or channels of light as shown in figure 10.1 (and Plate I).

Say the mantra *om* either silently or out loud: *ohhh* as the energy is rising and *mmm* as it is spiraling downward. Visualize the ascending golden light in the central channel and the golden fountain spiraling down and all around the subtle body, creating the form of a tube torus.

❀ Third Movement—Seven Multidimensional Chakras

The energy is next visualized rising up through each of the seven chakras, with any amount of detail as to the qualities and associations of each chakra (see examples below). Combine this visualization while applying the *mula bandha*— tightening the anal sphincter as you inhale to move the energy up to the next ascending chakra. Ending at the crown chakra, place the left hand very gently on the top back of the skull and experience the subtle energy above the top of the head.

❀ Fourth Movement—Centering

This movement brings the energy into the area of the heart, the central chakra, for meditation from the top down and the bottom up. Placing the tongue against the roof of the mouth, bring the united energy down from the crown chakra and then the Ajna chakra via the mantra meant for connecting the head to the heart via the throat, *aing hung aing*. Repeat at least three times.

Next, visualize the energy moving up from the root center to the heart center. This time move it deeper inward toward the central bindu of each of the first four chakras while emphasizing the outer planets—Uranus, Neptune, Pluto, and Eris. Move the energy to the heart center where we complete the meditation from this central bindu in the subtle body center, as presented below.

Mantras of the Lower Four Chakras

Utilize the four following mantras or chants while raising the energy through the central dot, or bindu, of the lower four chakras:

Root chakra: gayatri mantra (*om bhur bhuvah svah, tat savitur varenyam, bhargo devasya dhimahi, dhiyo yo nah prachodayat*) (Adoration of the Supreme Being.)

Sacral chakra: *om ganga yamuna saraswatiay namaha* (Adoration of the three sacred rivers of India. Three of your favorite rivers can be substituted.)

Navel chakra: *om mani padme hung* (Praise to the Jewel in the Lotus.)

Heart chakra: On the exhale, chant *gate gate paragate parasamgate bodhi swaha* (gone, gone, completely gone, absolutely totally gone, awake!). Silently on the inhale, *om*.

Once the energy is folded into the central point in the heart chakra from both the upper and lower three chakras, focusing on the breath in the central chakra can be with natural breathing or with an emphasis on the inhale breath as bringing in refreshing life and the exhale as the dissolution of all separation. This central meditation can begin with Baba Hari Dass's twenty-four hand mudras and end with his eight hand mudras. (For more information about these mudras, see *Ashtanga Yoga Primer*.)

✦✦✦

The first part of the contemplation through the signs of the zodiac can be seen as circular. Although the ida and pingala nadis are often shown as spiraling snake-like around the central sushumna nadi, in this meditation, the circular path is followed.

The second part of the contemplation involves inhaling up the straight central tube, while the fountain spraying out the top of the crown chakra and down around the whole subtle body creates the shape of a tube torus along with two intertwining channels of light.

There are many ways to do the third method, including the examples in the next section. Be creative.

Finally, the path inward through the first four chakras toward the central bindu in the heart center might be visualized as approaching a black or white hole in the center of each of the four lower chakras while going in deeper and deeper. When focusing on the breath, inhale with the mantra *om* and exhale with the heart sutra mantra of *gate gate paragate parasamgate bodhi swaha,* the mantra of no self.

ASTROYOGA CHAKRA MEDITATION

The following are some hints as to a routine that I use either along with the above contemplation or by itself; however, each practitioner will hopefully be creative about using the asanas, visualizations, and so on according to her or his particular practice.

Note that the seed mantras of the chakras have a nasal quality that is meant to have a strong vibratory effect on the head and the nasal and third-eye area. I visualize simple images of the seven chakras; although if you prefer, there are many available images of the chakras that are much more complex, with animals, divinities, objects, and so on. Often feminine angels or goddesses called dakinis are associated with the seven chakras. Below are examples of dakinis or goddesses that I find are attuned with the chakras; however, it might be more helpful to use images that are personally resonant for you.

First Chakra

Visualize the Muladhara chakra, a red four-petaled lotus with a golden square, in the tailbone area of the body. Asana: seated forward bend variations (*paschimottanasana*). Visualize the kundalini serpent coiled around the Shiva lingam, awakening with a hissing sound. On the upward ida side, focus on the sign of Aquarius. On the downward side, focus on the sign Capricorn.

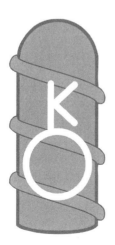

Fig. 10.2. Kundalini lingam with the sign of Chiron

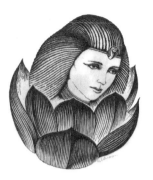

Fig. 10.3. *Egypt Lotus Queen*
by Bruce Harman

Dark goddess: earth dakini, mantra: *lang lakiniye namaha*. The dakini of the first chakra can be asked for assistance in feeling satisfied and complete with the material world and finances—safe and prosperous.

Second Chakra

Visualize the svadhishthana chakra, an orange six-petaled lotus with a silver crescent, in the sacral area. Asana: butterfly pose (*bhadrasana*). Visualize a silvery crescent Moon like a bowl filling with white lunar fluid. The upward sign Pisces is attuned to this sacral center. On the downward side, focus on Sagittarius.

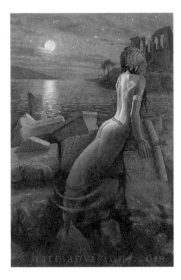

Fig. 10.4. *Mermaid Nocturne*
by Bruce Harman

Water dakini, mantra: *vang vakiniye namaha*. The dakini of the second chakra can be asked for help feeling satisfied and fulfilled in relation to emotional stability, reproduction, and pleasure.

Third Chakra

Visualize the Manipura chakra, a yellow ten-petaled lotus with a fiery red triangle, in the navel area. Asana: thunderbolt pose (*vajrasana*). Visualize fire being circulated throughout the subtle body. Focus on the fiery sign Aries on the upward path and intense sign Scorpio on the downward side.

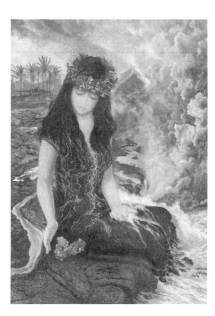

Fig. 10.5. *Pele*
by Bruce Harman

Pele: fire dakini, mantra: *rang rakiniye namaha*. The dakini of the third chakra can be asked to assist in feeling complete about issues related to fame, power, and control, including feeling well fed, nourished, and comfortable temperature-wise.

Fourth Chakra

Visualize the Anahata chakra, a green twelve-petaled lotus with a green six-pointed star, in the heart center filled with love for all beings. Asana: squatting balance poses (*vakasana, padangusthasana*) or seated spinal twist (*matsyendrasana*); mantra: *yang*. Visualize love radiating out from the heart. The upward sign Vacca/Taurus is associated with this center, as is the downward sign Libra.

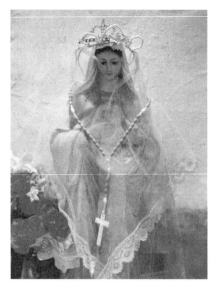

Fig. 10.6. Mother Mary,
photo courtesy
Sherry Burkart

Mother Mary: air dakini, mantra: *yang yakiniye namaha*. The dakini of the fourth chakra can be consulted for her help with feeling satisfied and complete about love, intimacy, and relationships.

Fifth Chakra

Visualize the Vishuddha chakra, a blue sixteen-petaled lotus, in the area of the throat. Asanas: seated backward bend or camel pose (*ushtrasana*), shoulder stand (*sarvangasana*), or fish pose (*matsyasana*). Visualize a sparkling blue sphere in the throat communicating truth. Gemini is the upward sign related to this center. Virgo is the sign on the downward pingala path.

Yeshe Chogal: ether dakini, mantra: *hang hakiniye namaha*. The dakini of the fifth chakra can be called on to feel satisfied and complete about communication skills and abilities to perceive subtle messages.

Sixth Chakra

Visualize the Ajna chakra, a blue-violet or white two-petaled lotus, in the middle of the forehead or third eye. Asanas: child's pose (*balasana*) or lotus pose (*padmasana*) with forehead to the floor. Visualize the

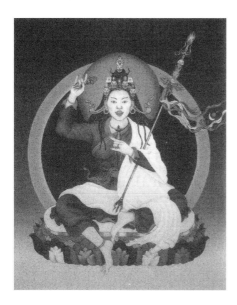

Fig. 10.7. Yeshe Chogal

skull as a bell and the two petals of the Ajna chakra as the wings of a white awakened dove or swan flying upward. The sign Cancer goes with this center.

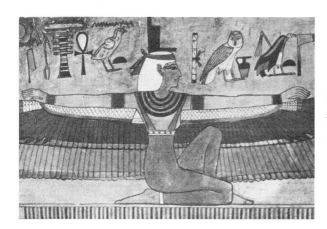

Fig. 10.8. Isis, from the tomb of Seti I, 1360 BCE

Isis: sound dakini, mantra: *tang takiniye namaha.* The dakini of the sixth chakra can be asked for assistance in feeling that the mind is calm, clear, and peaceful. She can also be called on for help with musical abilities.

Seventh Chakra

Visualize the Sahasrara chakra, a multicolored multipetaled lotus, in the area at the top of the head. Asanas: headstand (*shirshasana*) or dolphin pose (*padmasana*) and then liberation pose (*muktasana*). The mantra *ham-sa* (I am that) is appropriate with the upward ida side, *so-ham* (That I am) with the pingala side, and then *om* (the sound of creation or before, beyond the separate self). With the *ohhh*, visualize the energy rising up the central sushumna channel to the thousand-petaled lotus on top of the skull. Visualize golden light penetrating the central bindu of this chakra and streaming out the top like a fountain. Golden mist from the fountain can pour down over the subtle body with the *mmm*. Leo is the sign of the zodiac associated with the crown chakra.

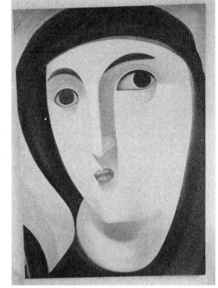

Fig. 10.9. *Sophia* by Prasanna

Sophia, mantra: *dang dakiniye namaha*. The dakini of the seventh chakra can be called on for help in letting go of the illusion of the separate self.

At the top of the head, the royal union of the Sun and Moon can be celebrated (perhaps visualizing a beautiful annular solar eclipse

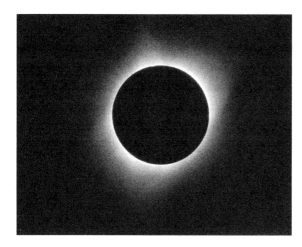

Fig. 10.10. Eclipse,
image from NASA

or the Tibetan *yab-yum* image) and then one can either continue meditating here or return back to the root center and from there on to a focus on the heart center using the AstroYoga techniques above.

Finally, with or without a mantra, focus on the breath: with each inhalation, watch the mind create the world of name and form, and with each exhalation, watch everything, including especially the illusion of a separate self, dissolve.

Meditation can end with a bow and beaming love to all, followed by the corpse pose (*savasana*). Of course, once again, all these directions are open to modifying the process with what feels right and with inspiration from the now. *Namaste!*

PART 3

✦ ✦ ✦

EXPLORING ASTROLOGICAL EVENTS

11

Introduction to
Chart Interpretation

In the next chapters, we will discuss practical examples of how the Alchemical Tantric Arrangement can illuminate deeper meaning when paired with a traditional astrology chart. We'll begin with some easy steps to interpreting a standard Western astrological chart and detail the differences with the Hermetic Chart. Remember, you can always look back to chapters 1 and 2 for more information about each sign's symbols, ruling planet, element, and other features.

1. **Sign and planet symbols.** First, get acquainted with the symbols for the signs and planets.
2. **Orientation.** Get oriented with the chart's basic directions. The top of a standard Western chart is oriented to the south, making the left side the east; the bottom, north; and the right side, west. This is because in the Northern Hemisphere, as we look toward the Sun, Moon, and planets in the sky, they appear to rise on our left, reach their highest point in the south, and set in the west, to our right. The twelve signs and houses start on the left side of the chart and proceed down and around the wheel counterclockwise.
3. **Key components.** Locate the Sun, Moon, and ascendant, or rising (easternmost), sign. Note the signs of the zodiac in which they are located. They are the three most important parts of the chart.

The Sun tells about the yearly cycle, the Moon about the monthly cycle, and the ascendant, the daily cycle. You are probably already acquainted with the meaning of these three components or you can look them up in this book.

4. **Chart geometry.** Next, look at the overall shape of the chart to determine if there are obvious collections of planets around the wheel. This is a way to discover areas of the chart and planets that are accented.

5. **Ruling Planets.** Another way to determine which planets are accented is to identify the ruling planets of the signs that are located in the Sun, Moon, ascendant, and collections of planets. You can look up planetary rulers of the signs in this book or easily on line.

6. **Elements and aspects.** Two more ways to find the more highlighted parts of a chart involve finding the element of each accented sign and also looking at the planets with the largest number of lines connecting them to other planets. These lines that are usually colored on the charts indicate the angular relationship between the planets and are called aspects. Once again you can find the element, earth, water, fire, or air, of any sign in this book.

Here is a chart of the most important aspects and their meaning.

CHART ASPECTS AND RELATIONSHIPS

NAME	COLOR	ANGLE	MEANING
Conjunction	–	0 degrees	sharing energy
Semi-sextile	orange	30 degrees	differing views
Sextile	green	60 degrees	good sharing
Square	red	90 degrees	difficult side issues
Trine	blue	120 degrees	most harmonious
Inconjunct	brown	150 degrees	tension
Opposition	red	180 degrees	opposing views

164 * Exploring Astrological Events

7. **Integration.** Then the fun begins: integrating all the information discovered from reading about the most highly accented signs and planets to come up with an overall picture or composite story of the particular individual or event.

8. **Transits.** Determining the most accented signs and planets in an astrological chart, as we did above, is also an important step in the process of following the timing of transits or where the planets are presently moving. For example, if you discovered that your Sun, Moon, or ascendant is in the sign of Capricorn, because there have been so many important planets transiting through this sign recently, you can be certain that these last few years have been especially intense for you, and major shifts to noticeably different feelings and themes can be expected as planets transit into the next sign of Aquarius. This particular transit from Capricorn to Aquarius is noteworthy because it is accented in Alchemical Tantric Astrology.

INTERPRETING THE ALCHEMICAL TANTRIC ARRANGEMENT CHART

1. Orienting to the Hermetic (ATA) chart is easier because it is based on a relationship of the twelve signs and their ruling planets to the seven chakras, which means that every Hermetic chart starts with the same format. Every Hermetic chart, will always have the same sign correspond to the same chakra; for example, everyone's Cancer planets will be placed next to the sixth, or Ajna, chakra. You can use the ATA with numbered houses or a copy of plate 1 to expand and enter your planetary data.

2. The Hermetic chart begins at the bottom right with the sign Aquarius next to the first, or root, chakra and ascends counterclockwise through the zodiac and chakras in their usual order. Upon reaching the sign of Leo in the crown chakra, the signs continue through the zodiac back down the chakras to Capricorn and the first, or root, chakra.

3. I have written out the names of the planets in the Hermetic chart rather than use astrological symbols. All the planets (including the ascendant) from the standard Western astrology chart are entered next to their corresponding sign and chakra in the Hermetic chart.

4. Interpretation involves looking at which planets and how many are related to which chakras. The correspondences developed in this book, with this new arrangement of the zodiac and the addition of chakras and alchemical metals, adds more developed symbolism and meaning to the standard astrological chart.

5. For examples of how the Hermetic chart was developed and for comparisons between standard charts and Hermetic charts, see chapter 12.

The Sun, Moon, and all the planets make their journeys through the zodiac (transits) and can be seen as carriers of their particular light and energy obtained through an alchemical, kundalini process as they pass through the cycle of signs. Of course, each planet moves at its own pace, depending on the duration of its cycle. For example, the Moon takes a month to complete its cycle through the zodiac, while Pluto takes approximately 250 years. We can attune to this alchemical, tantric process by being aware of the planetary transits through the various signs and chakras and thereby utilize the subtle assistance of each of their energies.

Although each planet and sign has its part to play in the grand celestial drama, this arrangement (ATA) of the zodiac, which places Capricorn and Aquarius at the bottom and first, or root, chakra with Cancer and Leo at the top and seventh, or crown, chakra, puts an extra emphasis on the ruling planets of these four signs: Saturn, Uranus, Moon, and Sun. Both Chiron and the nodes of the Moon are also accented. I suggest that these four planets, plus Chiron and the nodes, be given extra attention as they transit through the zodiac and also as they transit through a person's natal chart. The Sun and Moon will transit yearly and monthly through the complete zodiac. However, Saturn, Uranus, Chiron, and the nodes move more slowly, so their transits are rarer.

Barbara Hand Clow's book *Astrology and the Rising of Kundalini: The Transformative Power of Saturn, Chiron, and Uranus* also addresses the power of these outer bodies. Her emphasis is on the period of time between a person's first Saturn return, about age thirty, through the time when Uranus is opposite its natal position, age forty-two, and culminates at the person's Chiron return, about age fifty. It makes perfect sense to me that these three planets would be involved in the rising of kundalini around this time known as the midlife crisis.

12
Reading Key
Moments of the Past

It is a striking coincidence that the time period around 2020 contained transits of Saturn and the nodes over the pivotal cusp between Aquarius and Capricorn. Transits of the nodes of the Moon dramatically emphasized eclipses of the Sun and Moon. It is notable that all the outer radioactive planets have transited or will transit this sensitive cusp in order: Uranus transited in 1995, Neptune in 1998, and Pluto will transit in 2023–2024. Chiron transited into Aquarius in 2005, and Jupiter and Saturn were conjunct exactly on this potent portal at the end of 2020. After Pluto enters Aquarius to stay in 2024, every major planet from Jupiter to Eris will be on the upward activating, or accumulating, side of the Hermetic chart. This suggests an overall positive time, like the season of spring on a grand scale. (See chapter 13 for more information about transits through the ATA.)

What follows is an expanded version of the historical threads that are woven into the tapestry of ideas found in this book. It is an astrological journey following hints that presented themselves in a series of spontaneous initiations. The emphasis will be on interpreting the astrology of these events.

MESSENGER
FROM THE WATER GATE

Let's start a particular story I have alluded to in earlier chapters. It takes place in Santa Cruz (Holy Cross), California, where I helped with the construction of a large redwood labyrinth on the new campus of the University of California. This project, and my related studies, led me in a few directions.

The first life-changing result was meeting Himalayan master yogi Baba Hari Dass, which was the beginning of what has become a life-long yoga practice. It felt like building the labyrinth was an alchemical project. As soon as it was completed, a wonderful yoga teacher appeared.

A second result of building and studying the labyrinth was that it gave me the inspiration to travel with an aim to engage with archetypes around the world. This led me to explore labyrinths and power spots, and I visited such places as Stonehenge and the Parthenon, finally arriving in Knossos, Crete, site of the famous labyrinth and site of the original myth of the Minotaur. Next on my itinerary was to visit the Great Pyramids in Egypt.

However, this was October of 1973 and a war suddenly broke out in the Middle East. I could no longer travel by ship from Crete to Alexandria. So I traded my ticket to Egypt for passage on a ship headed to Barcelona and the tiny Spanish island of Formentera, where I had learned a wise astrologer lived. And, indeed, I did meet this French astrologer, named Isong, exactly on my thirtieth (golden) birthday, October 30, 1973. As if expecting me, Isong invited me to stay in a cottage near his, where I was able to study books from his well-stocked library, with plenty of time to meditate.

A few months later, around Christmas 1973, an unusual experience tuned me into the "music of the spheres" and a series of related insights. It was this astonishing experience and my attempt to understand it that is at the basis of this book.

The sound began as a ringing in my ears, which at first I didn't pay much attention to because I had a persistent ringing following my experiences of being near explosions and big guns in Vietnam in 1969–1970. However, eventually the sound grew loud enough that I thought there must be a big generator running nearby on the little island of Formentera. I explored around the island but could not find the location of any external sound. Since the volume of sound remained constant, I had to consider that it must indeed be an inner sound.

It grew louder and more melodic until it was clearly more like music. Eventually, the sound took on more of the sound of Indian music, with a droning *om*-like background. Then singing voices appeared, and more instruments began to play. Over a period of about a week, the sound became so loud and constant that I was hardly able to sleep. It seemed that the full Mormon Tabernacle Choir and the New York Philharmonic Orchestra were in my little cottage. The voices appeared to be singing in some unknown language. Finally, I got so exhausted that I began to fear for my life or at least my sanity. Climbing up the highest hill near my cottage, I fell down on my knees and prayed for the volume to be turned down, and from that time on, it did indeed slowly subside. For a few weeks thereafter, every sound, even cars driving on the nearby road, seemed to mix together perfectly in an overall *om*-like sound.

Having a great interest in astrology, I started looking toward the heavens to see if I could understand more about what was happening from an astrological perspective. I discovered that this all coincided with the passage of Comet Kohoutek on Christmas eve near the time of a solar eclipse. I knew there was something special about this so I took these as amazing hints to help me understand my experience.

In the diagrams below (figures 12.1 and 12.2), note the comet's perigee (closest to Earth), which happened on December 21, 1973, on the winter solstice. Perihelion (closest to the Sun) occurred on December 27, forming a grand cross in the cardinal signs involving Saturn, Pluto, the Sun, the Moon, Eris, and Chiron, all planets that I now know are especially important in Hermetic astrology.

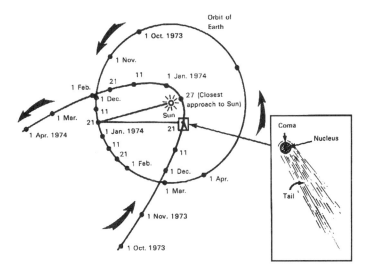

12.1. Comet Kohoutek perigee and perihelion, winter 1973

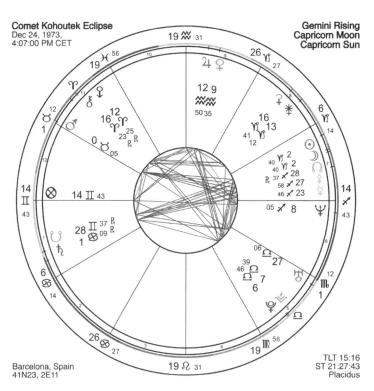

Fig. 12.2. Chart near winter solstice eclipse, December 24, 1973,
Comet Kohoutek eclipse

With Comet Kohoutek blazing overhead, I considered it to be a harbinger of events to come, like a torchbearer announcing the opening of of the Cosmic Olympics. Then, I started looking at the astrological charts of future alignments that might include similar patterns, especially ones that involved Capricorn and the other cardinal signs. Christmas Eve 1973, had been accompanied by a solar eclipse at 2 degrees of Capricorn, opposite Saturn retrograde at 1 degree of Cancer. The north node and Pallas were close to the degree of the Galactic Center. As might be expected from this portentous astrology, these were amazingly eventful times in other ways also, such as the war in Vietnam and the impeachment of Capricorn president Richard Nixon. In ancient times, it was generally thought that comets could spell disaster for the rulers of the realm!

THE GREAT 1989 ALIGNMENT

My time on Formentera with its heavenly concert was a wonderful Christmas gift from the cosmos with Comet Kohoutek as a cosmic messenger. Pondering Kohoutek's message, it appeared to be pointing ahead to the great Capricorn-Cancer alignment of the winter of 1989–1990 (see figure 12.3).

With a new Moon in Capricorn and all the planets opposing Jupiter retrograde in Cancer, the 1989–1990 alignment was certainly *the* alignment of the twentieth century! It did indeed turn out to be a very eventful time period, including, for example, the Valdez oil spill, the fall of the Berlin Wall, and the Santa Cruz, California, earthquake. Furthermore, as a continuation of this monumental alignment, in 1993 Uranus and Neptune came together to begin another once in a lifetime major cycle while still in the sign of Capricorn.

2010–2011: THE TOHOKU EARTHQUAKE AND TSUNAMI

The most massive planets in our solar system, Jupiter and Saturn, aligned in opposition during the time period around 2010–2011, square

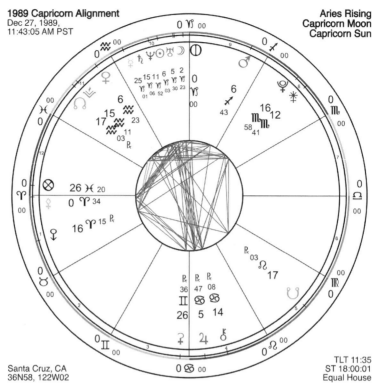

Fig. 12.3. Great Capricorn alignment
of December 27, 1989

to the solstice and Galactic Center axis. Although Jupiter had earlier transited the Galactic Center, by 2010 (figure 12.4).

Jupiter entered into the great T-square conjunct Uranus in Aries to oppose Saturn in Libra, forming the horizontal arms of the grand cross rather than the "vertical" axis of 1989–1990, when we experienced the strong earthquake in Santa Cruz, California.

The theory that earthquakes can be influenced by planetary alignment can be likened to the way that the moon contributes to the highest tides. In this sense, the Jupiter effect may not have been as powerful in this particular opposition to Saturn as it was in 1989–1990, although the remainder of the factors certainly implied profound transformation. To have anticipated such transformation was hardly a prediction, given

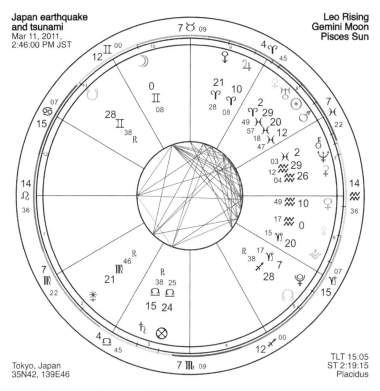

Japan earthquake
and tsunami
Mar 11, 2011,
2:46:00 PM JST

Leo Rising
Gemini Moon
Pisces Sun

Tokyo, Japan
35N42, 139E46

TLT 15:05
ST 2:19:15
Placidus

Fig. 12.4. Chart of Tohoku earthquake and tsunami,
March 11, 2011

the numerous indicators of massive change well under way at the time, and with the remainder of the melting iceberg of environmental, political, social, and personal transformation and/or disaster looming on the horizon.

In the case of the massive and ongoing devastation in Japan from the earthquake and tsunami of March 11, 2011, it appears that the geocentric opposition, in addition to the almost exact heliocentric opposition of Jupiter and Saturn, was a potent combination. Given the direct destruction from the earthquake and tsunami and the consequent Fukushima Daiichi nuclear disaster, I would say that this catastrophe qualifies as apocalyptic. The cardinal T-square involving Jupiter, Saturn, and Pluto was definitely a factor, as was the exact mutual reception of Uranus and Neptune at the end of Pisces and Aquarius.

2012 AND THE ENDING OF THE MAYAN LONG COUNT CALENDAR

There is speculation that the ancient Mayan astronomers chose the time period around 2012 to end their long count calendar because it coincides with the alignment of our winter solstice with the Galactic Center, the dark rift near the central bulge in the Milky Way. The Mayan Long Count Calendar covers approximately one-fifth of the 26,000-year cycle related to the precession of the solstice and equinox points, due to the slow wobble of Earth's north pole.

The ancient and present-day Maya view the cross as representing the intersection of our Milky Way Galaxy with the ecliptic. The symbol of the cross of the four cardinal signs, or directions, drawn within the circle is found in many cultures worldwide and, in fact, is used as a symbol to represent planet Earth.

As mentioned above, there is evidence that the Maya were pointing toward the winter solstice of 2012 because it is part of the larger cosmic cycle related to the precession of the equinoxes, the roughly 26,000-year great cycle. It is quite possible that the Maya wanted to draw our attention to the fact that this grand cycle has reached its equivalent of midwinter in our yearly cycle. When the winter solstice point of Capricorn aligns with the Galactic Center, our Sun is at the point farthest away

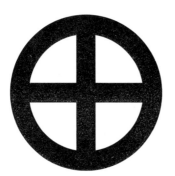

Fig. 12.5. The grand Galactic Cross

but still aligned with the center of our Milky Way Galaxy. It is a moment that, like the winter solstice, is at once the darkest time and, at the same time, is holding the seeds of the return of the light. Some have noted that the Vedic great ages, called yugas, may also be related to this precession cycle. If so, humanity could also be near the darkest point of the Kali Yuga and close to beginning the turn toward more enlightened ages for the next 12,000 years.

THE GRAND CROSS AND PATTERNS OF MAJOR SHIFTS

Major planetary alignments are not the only cause of large-scale shifts on the planet, but they can be important contributing factors. Indeed, the time period around 1989–1990, with its impressive alignment, did coincide with major earthquakes and many other significant shifts, including the fall of the Berlin Wall. Likewise, the huge Japanese earthquake and tsunami in 2011 involved an opposition of Jupiter and Saturn. What is most intriguing is that a pattern of celestial phenomena, demonstrated especially by these three cosmic events—the close approach of Comet Kohoutek to Earth and the Sun at Christmas 1973; the great alignment of 1989–1990 in Capricorn; and the grand squares of the period leading up to and including the end of the Mayan Long Count Calendar at the end of 2012—all point to the cardinal cross, the ancient spiritual symbol found in cultures worldwide and related in many ways to Christ, Christmas, and the winter solstice. That the ending of a major cycle of the Mayan Long Count Calendar corresponded to the alignment of this same Capricorn solstice with the Galactic Center is amazing, to say the least. Add to this the dwarf planet Pluto (divinity of the apocalypse) transiting the Galactic Center, eclipses along this same axis (note the added symbolism of the serpent or dragon related to the Moon's nodes), earthshaker and tsunami-maker Neptune entering his home sign of Pisces and—*wow!* The signs are indeed impressive.

Some folks say, "Nothing special happened in 2012." However,

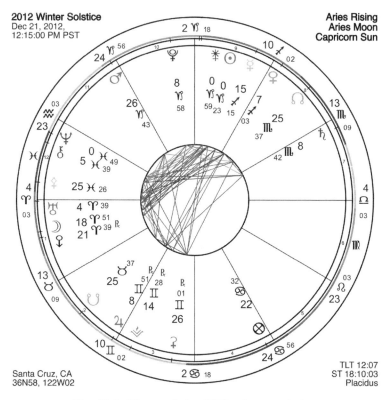

Fig. 12.6. Chart of the 2012 winter solstice,
December 21, 2012

I think that we could find quite a few rather major events to the contrary. Just before midnight of New Year 2012, President Barack Obama, despite being a constitutional lawyer, signed into law the National Defense Authorization Act, which included the draconian provision for unlimited military detention of American citizens without due process of law, adding another nail in the Kali Yuga coffin of 2012. New Year's Eve represents the extremes of the darkest night and the rebirth of the light and is once again strongly connected to the midwinter symbolism of Capricorn. It was also in 2012 that the ecological calamity of global climate change, which had been approaching for some time, became shockingly obvious.

2012 TO NOW

Although the powerful square among the intense actors, apocalyptic Pluto in Capricorn and radical Uranus and Eris in Aries, continued through this time period, the energetic effects seemed to become even more magnified when Jupiter entered Libra in 2016, adding another arm to the T-square, especially with surprising Uranus moving closer to chaotic Eris in fiery Aries. It would appear that the Trump phenomenon is largely related to this powerful cardinal formation. President Donald Trump's inauguration exactly on the potent Chiron portal, and the dramatic Women's March that followed on January 21, 2017, the day after the inauguration, stirred up huge emotional responses around the world.

President Trump's persona and actions have had the earmarks of the Uranus-Eris conjunction in Aries, with all the division and turmoil of shock, reaction, and resistance. President Trump continually brought drama onto the stage during his term of office. Of course, one particularly charged "apple of contention" was the perceived attempt of his administration to outlaw abortion. The "warrior woman" or "lover of justice" archetype, related to dwarf planet Eris, brought millions of women and men into the streets during his administration, not just after his inauguration but in racial justice protests during the 2020 election year.

Note in the chart in figure 12.7 how the Trump inauguration Sun landed exactly on the Chiron portal of 0 degrees Aquarius. Based on what we now know about the potency of the Chiron portal, there is no doubt that formidable energies for both revolution and evolution were activated.

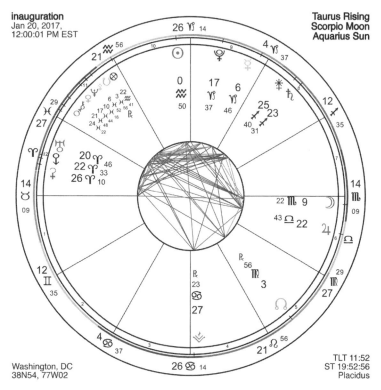

Fig. 12.7. Chart of President Trump's inauguration,
January 20, 2017

2017 TOTAL SOLAR ECLIPSE AND
2018 TOTAL LUNAR ECLIPSE

Also note the chart of the total solar eclipse that transited the entire width of the United States on August 21, 2017, at the end of dramatic Leo. It included yet another grand cross in the cardinal signs, although the square between Uranus and Pluto was moving farther apart.

This was clearly an important event for the entire country, as huge crowds all across the United States made their way under the path of totality for a dose of celestial wonderment. From the standpoint of Hermetic astrology, many noteworthy aspects accented Saturn, Uranus, Chiron, and the Moon's nodes, all rulers of the Hermetic chart.

As demonstrated more fully in the following section ("Transits of Rahu and Ketu"), it is particularly noteworthy to watch the transits of the Moon's nodes. Their placement near the vertical axis of hermetic charts has often turned up at pivotal times. When they move over charged parts of the Hermetic chart, such as the central axis of Leo-Cancer and Aquarius-Capricorn, they bring formidable eclipses to bear on the alignments, as shown in the charts in figures 12.8, 12.9, and 12.10. I have tracked their 18.5-year cycle, starting with my birthday in 1943 (see my birth chart, figure 12.15), where they fall appropriately at the top and bottom of the Hermetic chart, in Leo (Rahu) and Aquarius (Ketu). They return to this position again in 1962, 1981, 2000, 2018, and 2037.

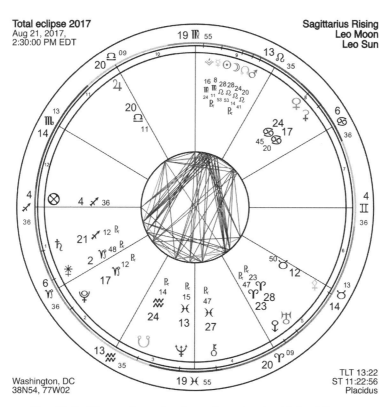

Fig. 12.8. Chart of total solar eclipse in the United States,
August 21, 2017

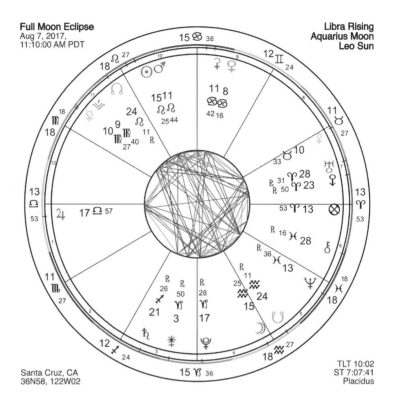

Fig. 12.9. Chart of Leo-Aquarius total full Moon eclipse near the Capricorn-Aquarius portal on August 7, 2017

Although the total eclipse of the Moon on July 27, 2018, was not as dramatic for the United States as was the total solar eclipse in Leo during 2017, in terms of the Hermetic chart, it is impressive how closely the Sun and Moon conjunct both the nodes and the Chiron-kundalini portal on the cusp of Aquarius and Capricorn.

Looking at former transits of the nodes over the central axis of the Hermetic chart has resulted in correlations with highly energetic events. The most monumental was the transit of the south node through Aquarius when the atomic bomb was actively being tested in 1944, and the terrible destruction unleashed when two bombs were detonated over Japan in 1945, when the south node had moved into Capricorn. The historical record suggests that powerful, radioactive,

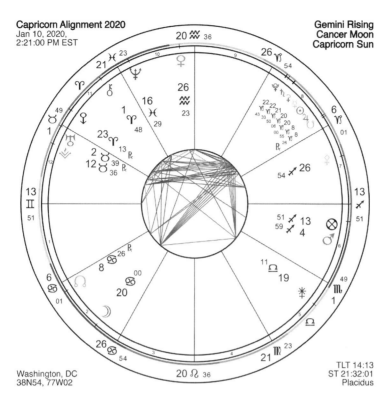

Fig. 12.10. Chart of impressive full Moon opposite Capricorn stellium on January 10, 2020. Notice the amazing grand cross in the cardinal signs correlated with the COVID-19 virus outbreak.

and evolutionary kundalini energy is awakened when the nodes are transiting Leo (Rahu) and Aquarius (Ketu), and the energy is used or abused as the nodes transit into Cancer and Capricorn.

The nodes entered Cancer-Capricorn at the end of 2018 and transited across a long line of planets in Capricorn during 2019 and into 2020, as shown in spectacular fashion in figure 12.10. It is especially clear now that we could have expected some major awakening and everything that follows. Of course this time correlates perfectly with the worldwide COVID-19 phenomenon. In the outer world, it continues to look ominous, and on the individual level, it depends on how we treat Ms. Kundalini and how she treats us! And everyone's personal astrology has a role to play!

TRANSITS OF RAHU AND KETU, THE NORTH AND SOUTH NODES OF THE MOON

As noted in chapter 2, Rahu and Ketu, also known as the head and tail of the dragon, have an important role to play in Hermetic astrology because of their symbolic connection as serpentine dragon to the serpentine kundalini.

The south node (SN) reached the exact potent portal between Aquarius and Capricorn on May 10, 1944 (see figure 12.11a). At that time the north node (NN) was between Mars in Cancer and Pluto in Leo. There was experimentation with building the atomic bomb at this time during World War 2. It was, of course, an extremely major and tragic event in human history when the first atomic bombs were dropped on highly populated cities in Japan in 1945. At that time, the SN was in Capricorn.

The SN was at 0 degree Aquarius on December 22, 1962, near to Saturn in Aquarius (see figure 12.11b). At this time during the Vietnam undeclared war, the Cuban missile crisis occurred. JFK was assassinated in 1963 with the SN in Capricorn.

On September 19, 1981, the NN was at 0 degree Leo near Mars in Leo (see figure 12.11c). In this year Ronald Reagan became president, Pope John Paul II was shot, the AIDS epidemic began, and IBM introduced its first personal computer. In 1982, with the SN in Capricorn, President Reagan declared a "war on drugs," the Falklands War was waged, and Israel invaded Lebanon.

The year 2000 came with its share of angst (remember Y2K?), and when the SN was at 0 degree Aquarius on April 8, 2000, Neptune was nearby in Aquarius and Pallas was near the NN in Leo (see figure 12.11d). September 11, 2001, the fall of the twin towers, occurred with the SN in Capricorn conjunct Mars.

The SN was retrograding through Aquarius during most of the year 2017 and crossed the 0 degree portal on November 6, 2018 (see figure 12.11e). Of course, we had President Trump, huge storms, and

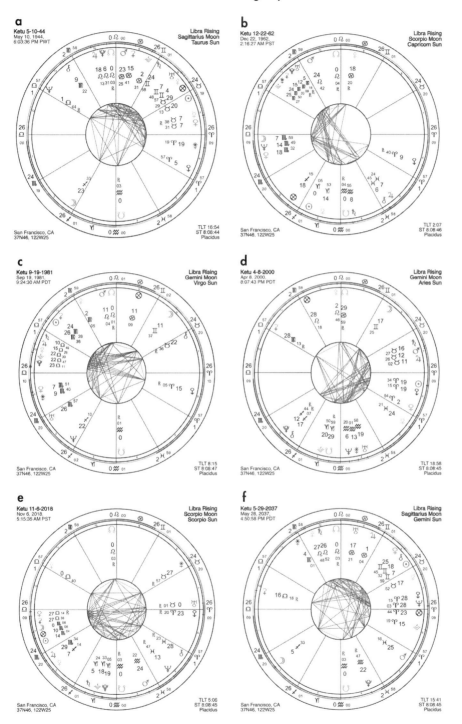

Fig. 12.11 (a–f). Six transits of Ketu

a continuation of war in the Middle East. In 2019 and 2020, the SN transited over Pluto and a long line of planets in Capricorn. Based on the advent of the coronavirus pandemic that shut down the whole world, I would say that it was a dramatic demonstration of the SN transiting not only Capricorn but also ten of the sixteen most active planets and asteroids.

May 29, 2037, will be the day of the next transit of the nodes through the portal or axis of Aquarius-Leo (see figure 12.11f). Along the way, 2036 will see the nodes transiting the always interesting opposition of Saturn and Pluto (remember 2001?), in this case in the hermetically charged signs of Aquarius and Leo. At the same time, Neptune will be conjunct Eris and Saturn will be conjunct Pallas. In 2038, with the SN transiting Capricorn and the NN transiting Uranus and Jupiter in Cancer, well—let's just hope that the humans make it that far!

Although intense events seem to be happening all the time lately, still it appears that eclipses happening near the radioactive kundalini axis of the Hermetic astrology chart activate the awakening of very powerful energy for good and not so good. Perhaps the clincher is the transit of the SN through Aquarius in 1776 for revolutionary fervor and into Capricorn and conjunct apocalyptic Pluto for the backlash from England and ensuing war.

20/20 VISION

Looking back at the year 2020, we experienced a major Capricorn alignment, with gigantic Jupiter and Saturn meeting apocalyptic Pluto. The year 2020 began with Pluto leading the celestial parade through Capricorn, followed by Saturn, Ceres, the Sun, the south node, Jupiter, and Mercury. The coronavirus started hitting the headlines on New Year 2020. Serious Saturn, being the ruling planet of Capricorn, apparently made Saturn especially influential. Then Saturn transitioned into Aquarius, retrograded, and did it all over again. The second time, old king Saturn and young king Jupiter crossed the threshold into Aquarius and ushered in the dawn of a new age together.

The grand alignment of Jupiter, Saturn, Pallas, and Pluto occurred near the critical cusp between Capricorn and Aquarius, followed by a change from the earth element into the quite different air element for Jupiter-Saturn conjunctions and the beginning of a new cycle of roughly two hundred years.

During 2020, there were dramatic eclipses and Mars transits through these same degrees of Capricorn, plus a plethora of major conjunctions, including the important conjunction of Jupiter and Saturn that was exact in the first degree of Aquarius at the end of 2020. This conjunction at the exact cusp between Capricorn and Aquarius, which can be considered the potent Chiron, or kundalini, portal, is monumental. The alignments of these two heavyweights of the solar system, Jupiter and Saturn, which have been occurring recently near the ten-year change of decades, has been correlated with major shifts on many levels, including earthquakes and radical social transformations. In terms of the alchemical and tantric potential, the opportunity for insights, evolution, and even recognition of oneness, is breathtaking.

LIGHT AND DARK: WINTER SOLSTICE 2020 AND BEYOND

I was expecting something major from this striking stellium in the final and profound sign in the Alchemical Tantric Arrangement when all the planets transitioned over the potent Chiron portal on the cusp of Capricorn and Aquarius. I did not imagine, however, the immense worldwide effects of the coronavirus pandemic. Could there be a more dramatic demonstration of the potential transformative power of an astrological point?

With the Trump wild card involved in a bizarre general election in the United States in November 2020 (read Scorpio), influential dwarf planet Pluto returning soon to its 1776 position and then transiting into Aquarius, along with the portentous meeting of the solar system heavyweights Jupiter and Saturn conjunct at 0 degrees of Aquarius, exactly on the potent portal . . . well, that's a deep subject. We can barely imagine what could possibly top what we have witnessed thus far with the whole world in lockdown, but the hits keep coming . . .

In many ways, the day of the Capricorn solstice at the end of 2020 was the astrological culmination of my investigating and writing this book. Starting with the amazing creation of the Santa Cruz labyrinth, which led me to the great labyrinth at Knossos, back to the heavenly choirs in Formentera at Christmastime 1973, and during all the "cosmic crosses," I was seemingly offered hints as to the importance of the Capricorn-Aquarius cusp in the Alchemical Tantric Arrangement of the signs of the zodiac.

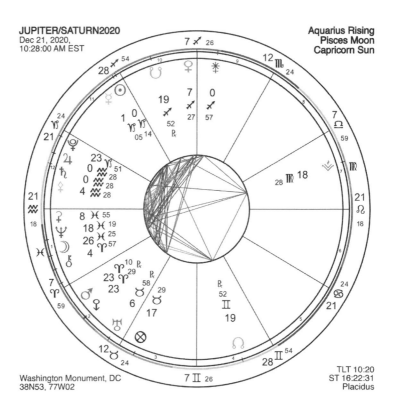

Fig. 12.12. Chart of the winter solstice, December 21, 2020, when Jupiter and Saturn were conjunct at the Chiron portal, 0 degree Aquarius, with Mars conjunct Eris and exactly square Pluto, plus Neptune opposite Vesta and square the nodes

This particular culmination in 2020 shown in figure 12.12 is once again like the 2012 ending of the Mayan Long Count Calendar, coming on the winter solstice, both a major completion and a stunning new awakening. Capricorn suggests the dark night of the soul, Aquarius the bright new day of the awakening spirit. The many prominent hard squares versus harmonious trines and the resonant polarity between mighty Neptune in his favorite sign, Pisces, exactly opposite sacred Vesta in appropriate Virgo, Uranus the awakener in Gaia's sign of steady Vacca/Taurus, all speak to this grand duality.

DOING OUR PART: THE EPIPHANY

There are clearly dark aspects to the cosmic cross and its Capricorn midwinter symbolism. However, if, in fact, the alignment of the winter solstice with the Galactic Center produces or acts as a conduit for major pulses of energy from this powerful core of our home galaxy, where our little planet is rocked in its spiral arms, then it can be envisioned as sending us milky (gala) nourishment for our development, both planetary and individually. No matter how literal this energizing flow, it still is prudent for us to do our part as good recipients. One of the best ways we can prepare for receiving the energetic blessing of these times is to use what I have called the Alchemical Tantric Arrangement (ATA) of the signs of the zodiac, which is described in this book, to focus our attention on optimal times and symbols. The visualizations and meditations of AstroYoga, suggested earlier, are also a good way to tune in to the message from the Great Central Gal (as in gal-axy).

Let us note that on the twelfth (read zodiac) day after Christmas on January 6 (read mid-Capricorn) comes the day of Epiphany, which is associated with the magi (read astrologers) discovering the Christ child and presenting their gifts including (alchemical) gold. We passed through another symbolically rich time, supercharged by a middle conjunction of Jupiter and Saturn in 2020 when they moved together into Aquarius, meaning that their conjunctions for many years will now occur in the air signs rather than the earth signs. Such a "middle conjunction" is associated with both Jesus and Muhammad.

The universal energy, represented by the massive black hole superstar at the center of our galaxy, appears to be offering us golden gifts that reveal the consciousness of the Christos, born in this lowly manger of the third planet from the Sun, to Earth Mother Gaia-Sophia, at this auspicious and portentous season. Is this one of the meanings of the dawning of the Age of Aquarius? The extremely close conjunction of Jupiter and Saturn, the likely "Christmas Star" of biblical fame coming as it does more than 2000 years after the birth of Jesus certainly locates us in the window of a new great age.

ASTROLOGY OF THE NEW MILLENNIUM

Since we are speaking of new ages, let's backtrack slightly to another massive shift: The first moment of the year 2000, shown in figure 12.13. This is an especially important chart because it represents the beginning of a new year, a new decade, a new millennium, and a new great age of two thousand plus years. We'll reflect on the lessons developed thus far as we look at both the natural and Hermetic charts for this special moment.

Natural Astrology Chart of New Year 2000

The Sun, of course, is in the sign Capricorn, and at the bottom of the chart at midnight, trine to Saturn in Vacca/Taurus, square to Mother Ceres in balanced Libra, and sextile to the waning Moon in Scorpio. The New Year's astrological chart for midnight will always have the Sun around 10 degrees of Capricorn at the nadir. As noted earlier, I call this the Morpheus point because the midnight time near midwinter has affinities with the mythology of the divinity of dreams, sleep, and metamorphosis. It is instructive to be aware of the transits over this point.

In this very important chart, note that faithful Juno, queen of the divinities, and Mercury, guide of souls to the underworld, are close to the Morpheus point, also in Capricorn. Around the time of the great stel-

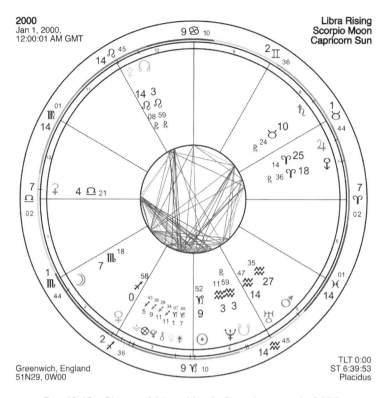

2000
Jan 1, 2000,
12:00:01 AM GMT

Libra Rising
Scorpio Moon
Capricorn Sun

Greenwich, England
51N29, 0W00

TLT 0:00
ST 6:39:53
Placidus

Fig. 12.13. Chart of New Year's Day, January 1, 2000,
Greenwich Mean Time

lium in Capricorn at the end of 1989, nebulous Neptune was right on this Morpheus point, and serious Saturn and surprising Uranus followed in the years soon after. Recently, apocalyptic Pluto has been transiting this portentous point (coming very close to conjunct in 2011, in time for the Tohoku earthquake and tsunami and Mayan Long Count end date).

The Moon is a waning Moon, falling in mysterious Scorpio, forming a positive sextile to the Sun and part of a rigid grand cross in the fixed signs. Waning Luna is challenged by all the squares but supported by ample earth signs, implying that the feminine is old, wise, and deep, and reminding us of Grandmother Hecate and Queen Persephone. Found in the second house, Lady Luna speaks about material issues in opposition or coordination with conservative Saturn retrograde in earthy Vacca/Taurus.

Mercury is ponderous in the sign Capricorn but helped along in conjunction with Queen Juno and the midnight Sun. Mercury gets different messages from a square to Mother Ceres and sextile to Mother Moon. He is motivated along his journey through the zodiac by Jupiter and Mars, even though not in resonant signs. In this moment, he is in his comfortable third house alongside Pluto, reminding us of Mercury's role as psychopomp and emphasizing him as a practical communicator using multiple talents to carry the soul to Hades's realm and back.

Venus, always the ruler of the New Year chart, is at the beginning of intelligent and playful Sagittarius, sextile to Neptune in Aquarius and Mother Ceres in Libra. Fortunately, lovely Venus is supported by devoted goddesses, sacred Vesta and Mother Ceres, in fire and air. Neptune is also helpful as a higher octave of Venus. Neptune conjunct the south node sets a spiritual and soulful tone to the eclipse cycle with an emphasis on surrender. Beautiful ruling Venus also tunes into the nodal axis harmoniously—great for connecting with the past and future, appropriate for the turn of the millennium.

Mars in Aquarius is sextile to Jupiter in Aries. They can work together for creativity and relationship, perhaps pulling and pushing erratic middle sister Eris into her higher octave. Mighty Mars is also sextile to Mercury, an odd couple, working together with mind and brawn in each other's exaltation.

Dwarf planet Ceres and the asteroid goddesses, Pallas, Juno, and Vesta, play important roles in this chart, forming many vital aspects. Mother Ceres is on the harmonious Libra ascendant; wise and powerful Pallas in the elevated tenth house in fiery Leo is pivotal as a member of the grand trine and grand square; royal Juno is at home in Capricorn and partnered with the dark dedicated Sun; and fiery sacred Vesta is conjunct Venus in one direction and a sacred presence in the powerful group on her other side.

Jupiter is especially brash in Aries conjunct Eris and sextile to Mars. The fire is hopefully not too hot in this seventh house of important relationships, but they will no doubt become highly charged. Royal

Jupiter, face-to-face with cunning Eris, could be a harbinger of spectacular gender face-offs. Jupiter appears to be armed and dangerous, but Eris knows how to speak truth to power. Massive Jupiter is especially powerful as a representative of the Galactic Center and is moving towards a meeting with the old king and father, Saturn, himself no lightweight. Expansive Jupiter in fiery Aries meets contractive Saturn, whose retrograde turns him back into solid Vacca/Taurus.

Saturn, ruler of the midnight Capricorn Sun, is comfortable in Vacca/Taurus and is part of the fixed grand cross, opposite to the Moon, and in a lovely earth trine to the Sun and Juno. This is a good solid placement for Grandfather Saturn, although the eighth house and retrograde motion seem sure to accompany long-lasting karmic lessons and complexities.

Chiron, the wounded healer, is found in favorable Sagittarius, the sign of the centaur, and is exactly conjunct apocalyptic Pluto and trine-elevated Pallas. There is a definite emphasis on healing in this chart, and we need this, but don't forget the depths of the wounding. The quincunx with Chiron's father, Saturn, could point to a cooperative relationship, although it might include removing the arrows in addition to healing the wounds.

Enlivening Uranus is in his home sign, Aquarius, making him the sole dispositor of the chart and accented in the significant grand fixed cross. Standing at the midpoint of Aquarius, which is the subtle beginning of spring, and sextile to intense Pluto and Chiron, in this chart, Uranus is a definite activator of the potent Chiron portal and Promethean awakener of the serpent kundalini in the root chakra. This placement could point to the opening of the upward movement of the radioactive path, fueled by Uranus's alchemical metal, uranium. All three radioactive rulers, Uranus, Neptune, and Pluto, plus Chiron, the centaur guardian of the threshold, are awakening together here at the base of the millennial mandala or chart, as more fully demonstrated in the Alchemical Tantric Arrangement on page 193 (fig 12.14).

Neptune, also in Aquarius, is part of the fixed T-square and trine Ceres. The conjunction and opposition with the nodes make Neptune vital in letting go of old patterns that get in the way of awakening. Neptune's soulful emotional involvement in this Aquarian sign is key to a more integrated healing.

Pluto, ruler of the Moon's sign, is strong in Sagittarius, conjunct Chiron, trine Pallas, sextile Uranus, and quincunx Saturn.

Eris, longtime resident of Aries, is especially strong in this chart. She brings her feminine wiles to the angular seventh house vis-à-vis giant Jupiter.

As always, the New Year's chart is similar to the Alchemical Tantric Arrangement, since at midnight, the Capricorn Sun is at the nadir near 10 degrees. The bottom of this spectacular chart accents the second through fifth houses, related to the lower chakras in the ATA, with Jupiter and Saturn moving toward a conjunction and elevated. Pluto conjunct Chiron in Sagittarius is a strong message of radioactive fire and healing. The symbolic grand cross in fixed signs speaks of solid structure and rigidity. Cardinal signs are on the angles, as usual in the New Year chart, with Mother Ceres rising in harmonious Libra. The grand trine in fire indicates that there will be plenty of rigidity balanced by plenty of fiery activism.

Hermetic Astrology Chart of New Year 2000

This is a prime example of how the Hermetic chart can augment the natural astrological chart. The Hermetic chart demonstrates other potentials in this vital horoscope for the new millennium, revealing full cycles of experience with a spiritual evolutionary significance, demonstrated by Capricorn and Aquarius planets galore.

Upon reading the Hermetic signs and chakras we immediately observe Neptune, Ketu, Uranus, and Mars in animating Aquarius. The presence of the radioactive outer planets alongside this first chakra and first ATA sign offer us a high-voltage charge for awakening, especially with Neptune at the south node shaking things up.

We also find this chart reflecting powerful third-chakra energy, with Eris and giant Jupiter together in fiery Aries. Dedicated Saturn in lovely Vacca/Taurus points us toward a serious heart focus.

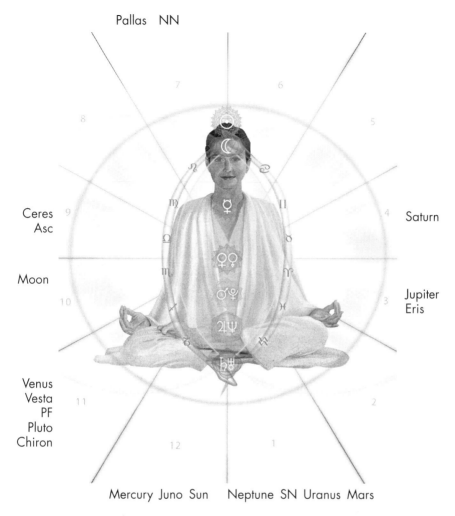

Fig. 12.14. Hermetic astrology chart of New Year 2000

Protective Pallas is in radiant Leo, crowning the caduceus, appropriately, with Rahu, the head of the dragon.

Moving down the chart to revisit the fourth chakra, we find Great Mother Ceres in artistic Libra, indicating the insights gained are beautifully expressed.

In the third chakra, notions of sacrifice are emphasized by the presence of the Moon in apocalyptic Scorpio.

In wise, fun-loving Sagittarius we have a full house. The chart's ruler, beautiful Venus, is alongside sacred Vesta and good fortune. We also find the exact conjunction of transformative Pluto and healing Chiron. It all points playfully to the delights of the second chakra.

Returning to the first chakra, we are greeted by Mercury, Juno, and the Sun in midwinter Capricorn!

This Hermetic chart especially accents the rich experience of Capricorn turning the corner past the kundalini energy of the potent Chiron portal into awakening Aquarius. Its immediate meeting with tsunami Neptune exactly conjunct the south node is a formidable indicator of shake-ups all across the board, at the beginning of the decade and beyond. Let's envision that the powerful awakening potential overcomes the current limitations of fear and uncertainty and that the promise of the great energy and unconditional love is fulfilled as in the image of protective Pallas at the crown chakra; that art, under the auspices of Mother Ceres, becomes the primary mode of expression; that the fear of death loses its sting with the help of lunar queen Persephone's awareness; and that we will begin the wise and playful Sagittarian celebration well before the end of the millennium.

ASTROLOGY CHART OF THE AUTHOR

The following are a few hints for those interested in my personal astrology. While reading books, I have often thought that it would be instructive to understand more about the author of the book via her or his astrology. So here goes . . .

Mercury accented. Mercury, ruler of my Virgo rising, with Mercury in the favorable third house and in a favorable air sign, Libra. Libra Mercury and Virgo Venus are in mutual reception.

Pluto accented. Pluto in Leo, ruler of the Sun and Moon in Scorpio, square to the Sun and in mutual reception.

Jupiter rising in Leo, quintile the Sun; conjunct ascendant and Regulus.

Chiron and Venus in the first house.

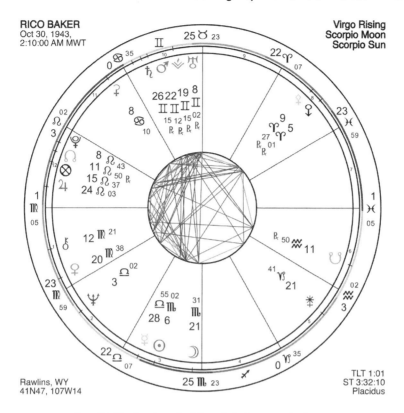

Fig. 12.15. Frederick "Rico" Baker natal chart

Alchemical arrangement with promethean Uranus at the midheaven inconjunct the Sun, with a bowl formation in the Eastern Hemisphere, ending with the royal alchemical marriage of Mercury, the Sun, and the Moon in the third house.

Head of the (kundalini uncoiled) dragon conjunct Pluto in Leo, with tail of the (kundalini coiled) dragon in Aquarius.

Eris and all the outer planets are accented. Eris is in T-square conjunct Pallas, square Ceres, and opposite Neptune. Eris is sextile Uranus, trine Pluto, widely inconjunct Chiron, and inconjunct Sun, so this forms a wide yod pointing at Eris in Aries (two inconjuncts with sextile in between create a thin triangle called a yod or a Finger of God because it looks like the triangle is a pointing finger).

There are also yods, or Fingers of God, from the Moon sextile Juno to Mars and Vesta, and another yod from the Sun sextile Chiron to Pallas (and widely Eris).

The quincunx or inconjunct I consider to be an "alchemical" aspect because its 150 degrees contains both the harmonious sextile and the stressful square. This combination, though not easy, is optimal for evolution because it contains both the challenge and the tools to overcome the challenge. The two planets of the sextile in a yod are especially helpful in working with the planet at the focal point.

There are seven quintiles, an aspect I especially enjoy since it involves segmenting the chart 72 degrees at a time. There is particular interest for me, since 72 is a multiple of 9, and the sum of single digits of any number that is a multiple of 9 equals 9. So 72 added together is 9 (7 + 2 = 9), as is 144 (1 + 4 + 4 = 9), 360 (3 + 6 + 0 = 9), and so on.

The seven quintiles within my own chart are between:

1. Sun and Jupiter
2. Moon and Chiron
3. Venus and Ceres
4. Mars and Pallas
5. Pluto and the midheaven
6. Vesta and the ascendant
7. Juno and Eris

AUTHOR'S
HERMETIC ASTROLOGY CHART

For comparison, the Hermetic chart is shown in figure 12.16. Everyone's basic Hermetic chart is the same, in terms of experiencing the same basic transits. Only the person's natal planets add the accents. This chart resembles the caduceus, the name of Hermes's herald staff, commonly depicted in the form of two serpents wrapped around a central rod, as is the tantric yoga subtle body image. In this version of the Hermetic chart, you can see that I have had the artist create the two snakes without spiraling to correspond more easily with the signs of the zodiac and their ruling planets.

You will see how my Hermetic astrology chart augments my natural astrology chart. The movement through the twelve Hermetic houses has the wonderful added benefit of being a complete spiritual tour up and down the seven chakras, seven alchemical metals, and seven traditional planets. The four "radioactive" planets and first four chakras lead directly into the heart center.

In the first Hermetic house of this Hermetic chart, we find the symbol for Ketu, the south node of the Moon (SN), in the sign of Aquarius. This is extremely fitting for the tail of the dragon to be found in the root chakra since it is where the coiled kundalini serpent is said to reside. As you'll recall, in Hindu myth, Ketu is the lower half of the demon who stole ambrosia from the gods and was then cut in two by Vishnu. Like Prometheus, Ketu represents a rebellious spirit who goes against the expected divine order. Thus radical, rebellious Ketu fits well with Aquarius and its ruling planet, Uranus. The nodes of the Moon are the points where new and full Moon eclipses occur and are especially accented times astrologically. In the year of my birth, 1943, eclipses occurred in Aquarius and Leo, giving special prominence to the main axis of my Hermetic chart.

One creation story related to the chakras says that the infinite energy of the universe comes down into the individual's body through the top of the head and is transformed down to each lower chakra from light to sound, then ether, air, fire, water, and finally compressed down into earth, coiled like a spring as the kundalini energy. Since universal energy is infinite, even this small portion is still infinite. The kundalini energy is coiled like a spring, primed for the return journey. This story is in keeping with the meaning of the south node as related to the past because it came from above and therefore the north node represents attraction back to the universal source.

The second house of my Hermetic chart, related to the second, or water, chakra and the sign of Pisces, does not contain any natal celestial

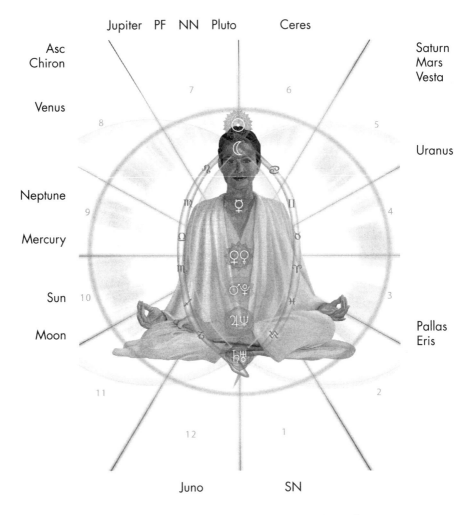

Fig. 12.16. Rico Baker's Hermetic astrology chart

objects. However, every transit through Pisces is activating this second chakra. Powerful Neptune, king of the sea and divinity of earthquake and tsunami, is presently residing here in the second chakra for us all. I imagine Neptune and his tantric partner, Salacia, embracing here, generating healing, loving energy.

The third Hermetic house is related to the third, or Manipura, chakra, which puts major emphasis on power and control. The dwarf planet Eris is located in my third Hermetic house in the sign of Aries.

Almost everyone alive has experienced this powerful influence, as challenging Eris has been in the sign of fiery Aries since 1927, and it will stay there until 2044. Eris appears to be prominent in the charts of those who have been mistreated or marginalized and are actively doing something about it.

All the world has been under the spell of this extreme placement of Eris in Aries for many years. This influence could easily be associated with all the wars of most of the twentieth century and the beginning of the twenty-first. We have had a particularly potent dose of Eris's energy, with the help of the recent transit of the Hermetic chart ruler, Uranus, over radically troublesome Eris. It is easy to associate the repeated conjunctions of these two problematic (but ultimately healing) planets with the surprising and radical time of the Trump era. During Trump's time in office as President, there was certainly ample focus on him via his domination of the media.

In mythology, Pallas is a fierce warrior goddess, so the fire of the sign Aries, along with the fire of the third chakra, emphasizes even more her dynamic warrior presence. Pallas Athene was the wise protector Goddess of ancient Athens, and in these times, I have experienced her as energizing my social activism. Having Pallas conjunct disturbing Eris natally can really stir the pot.

The fourth Hermetic house, related to the sign Vacca/Taurus and the fourth, or central, heart chakra, is not activated by any of my natal planets but has my midheaven here. Transits through Vacca/Taurus constellate a wide range of qualities represented by Venus/Aphrodite and Eris, cow and bull, earth and air, central one and sensual many. In terms of AstroYoga contemplation or meditation, it is helpful to focus on the rich sensuality of the love radiating heart along with the spiritual central heart. Until 2026, when Uranus enters Gemini, we will all have the mixed blessing of radical heavenly Uranus in relationship with his partner, Earth Mama Gaia. Theirs is both the primal union and the separation of heaven and earth, accented in the sign of the cow and bull.

The fifth Hermetic house makes up for the lack of natal planets in the fourth house with a natal stellium in the sign of Gemini. Two rulers of the Hermetic astrology chart, Saturn and Uranus, are both in this house along with Vesta, goddess of the sacred fire, and energetic Mars. The fifth Hermetic house is related to the fifth, or throat, chakra and the ether, or space, element. Communication is accentuated, and therefore Mercury, the divine herald and minister, is also evoked. Uranus, the radical innovator, initiates the far-reaching message, while Saturn, the conservative container, sets wise limits. This combination forms a rich alchemical image of the alembic, or pressure cooker, of transformation. Fiery Mars and Vesta provide their male and female forms of the heat and offer a tantric sexual element appropriate for the synergy of the fifth Hermetic house.

The sixth Hermetic house contains Ceres. In myth, she is the great Roman mother goddess, similar to Greek Demeter. This house relates to the sixth, or Ajna, chakra, located in the center of the forehead, and to the sign Cancer. The Moon is the ruling planet of Cancer, and the Moon's alchemical metal is silver. Ceres goes well with the symbolism of the silver queen, the powerful feminine presence of the all-seeing eye of intuitive wisdom and compassion.

On the cusp of the uppermost seventh Hermetic house, we come to the royal sign Leo, which is appropriately related to the crown chakra, the Sun, and the alchemical metal gold. The objects found here are Pluto, the north node, and Jupiter. Closest to this pinnacle is intense Pluto, ruler of my Sun and Moon's sign, Scorpio. The north node, or head of the dragon, is appropriately located at the top of the head and the crown chakra. Jupiter, king of the divinities, completes a formidable trinity comprised of heavenly father Jupiter; Rahu, kundalini risen, ruling the middle realms; and Pluto, king of the underworld.

In terms of the alchemical divine marriage, or hieros gamos, the two dwarf planets, Pluto in Leo and Ceres in Cancer, form the duality of underworld king and terrestrial queen. Their duality is also portrayed in the opposition of Pluto/Hades, the husband of Persephone, and Ceres/Demeter, the mother of the maiden Persephone. Royal golden Jupiter in Leo creates another duality with silvery Ceres in Cancer, as the marriage of heaven and earth.

The eighth Hermetic house contains my ascendant, healing Chiron and lovely Venus, all in Virgo, the healing sign of mutable earth. Quicksilver Mercury, the perfect guide down from the lofty heights and the ruler of Virgo and the fifth chakra, leads the downward distribution. Iris, the rainbow herald, is the feminine form of Mercury; hence, lovely Venus in this house, along with the beauty of the rainbow, leads the procession down the zodiac and chakras, with her beautiful presence and focus in Virgo on precise truth, to the next Hermetic house.

The two planets of the ninth Hermetic house, boundary-free Neptune and communicative Mercury, blend well with the feelings and meanings of Libra and the fourth chakra, the heart center. Neptune, as the higher octave of Venus, and Mercury/Hermes, the messenger, placed here on the axis of the grand cross, bring harmonious energy to Libra's emphasis on art and relationships.

The Sun and Moon, fresh from their new Moon union, both in the sign of Scorpio, offer their energy of new passionate starts and deadly endings. They are momentous participants in the third chakra's powerful energy and the tenth Hermetic house's fulfillment. The Sun illuminates and the Moon reflects their great radiance on themes of power, warmth, digestion, and penetration into hidden knowledge.

The eleventh Hermetic house, related to the sign Sagittarius, is without natal planets, as is Pisces, the other sign connected to the second, or sacral, chakra. This could suggest a lack of second chakra stimulation and my resultant desire to emphasize this chakra. Jupiter, representative of the Galactic Center and ruler of Sagittarius, recently transited this sign and Hermetic house, symbolically gearing up for his transit through busy Capricorn, where he brought his magnificent presence to the already monumental alignments of 2020.

Related to the twelfth and final Hermetic house and first, or root, chakra, this Hermetic house and sign of the fishgoat represents both the culmination of glory and the compost for the continuing cycles of life. Capricorn's alchemical metal, lead, can be seen as the heavy sinker. It is the alchemical prima materia that forms the basis of the alchemical process to transmute lead into gold.

Dedicated Juno, said in myth to be the queen of the divinities and wife to eminent Jupiter, king of the divinities, is quite comfortable here in the sign of Capricorn. Although she is powerful as the great mountain mother, Juno is also strong and confident enough to be the nurturing mother and wife.

Hopefully, this demonstrates how the Hermetic chart can spiritually augment the natural natal chart.

13
Looking Ahead
Major Future Transits of the Outer Planets

The Hermetic chart of ATA offers us a new handle on watching the movements of the planets with an eye toward their involvement in the spiritual development of individuals and the evolution of humanity. We can get a quick glance at this cycle of development toward alchemical and tantric union each month as the Moon moves to the top of the Hermetic chart in radiant Cancer and Leo. The resulting golden insights are showered down through the subtle body and integrated into our lives.

Similarly, each year shows us a full cycle of the Sun, Mercury, Venus, and half of a cycle of Mars. However we can get an especially good fix on our spiritual evolution by following Jupiter, a planet that stays one year in each sign and has recently begun its ascent through the ATA schema. Below we will look at some excellent hints about where we are heading as we follow transits through the ATA that all of us will be experiencing over the next few years.

TRANSITS OF JUPITER, SATURN, AND PLUTO

Mighty Jupiter will be fascinating to watch while this planet of expansion makes its way through the signs of the ATA. It passed through the potent Chiron Portal at the end of 2020, and between 2021 and 2026 it will move up through the seven ascending, accumulating signs of the ATA and their associated chakras, from Aquarius and the root chakra to Leo and the crown chakra. Along the way, Jupiter will be making conjunctions with all the outer planets: Jupiter was conjunct Pluto in Capricorn in 2020, Saturn at the beginning of Aquarius in late 2020, Neptune in Pisces in 2022, Chiron in Aries in 2023, Eris in Aries in 2023, and Uranus in Vacca/Taurus in 2024.

After Pluto enters Aquarius in 2023–2024, all of the outer planets will be on the ascending side of the alchemical, tantric system. This surely qualifies as one version of the dawning of the Age of Aquarius. Although this dawning has positive connotations, there will still be ample challenges in the so-called outer world. For example, technology will certainly continue to run amok. Across the board, we will likely see a perfect wave of apocalyptic changes all over the planet. Difficulties and challenges like the ones on the horizon, though not usually pleasant, often are helpful in the bigger picture when they spawn development of new abilities, creative solutions, and strong determination. As Friedrich Nietzsche said, "That which does not kill us, makes us stronger."

Pluto's upcoming transits are especially important because this divinity has daunting symbolism connected to the underworld and apocalyptic transformation. Before Pluto enters Aquarius to stay in 2024, it also returns to its position in the U.S. natal chart at 27 degrees of Capricorn. This is suggestive of a major death and rebirth for the United States.

When we look back half a cycle to the time Pluto last transited the Cancer-Leo cusp, it was in 1939—precisely the time of the beginning of World War II. We can certainly imagine Pluto's half-cycle fulfillment in many more positive ways than world war, but there is more than a hint of worldwide transition and turmoil suggested. Among other critical factors, the fallout from the coronavirus pandemic will certainly figure into this transition and turmoil.

In addition to all the intensity related to the Chiron/Kundalini portal, there is also the precedent of Pluto/Saturn conjunctions in Capricorn as being extraordinarily apocalyptic. This is likely related to Saturn's power in his home sign and the fact that both Saturn and Pluto have their south nodes in Capricorn, creating especially close alignments. (See Bruce Scofield's informative and relevant article, "Saturn Conjunct Pluto and the Return of Quetzalcoatl" in *The Mountain Astrologer,* June/July, 2019)

THE BIGGER PICTURE

It is tempting to interpret the movement of Jupiter suggested above as a major positive shift, from the darkness of midwinter Capricorn to the springtime awakening of Aquarius and upward through the ascending half of the zodiac and the related chakras. Indeed, Jupiter's expansive character will likely bring out more of the positive qualities of each of the conjunctions in their respective signs, houses, alchemical metals, and chakra associations. Each year after Jupiter has met with radical Uranus in 2024, he will continue moving upward through the signs, first through Gemini, the synthesizer, and then compassionate Cancer—where he is exalted—and then in 2026, wise radiant Leo at the crown chakra.

However, Pluto's apocalyptic effects in Capricorn have gone hand in hand with financial and social structural changes, and Jupiter seems to have added his weight to the intense Capricorn mix in the form of the coronavirus scare and financial apocalypse. This twelfth Hermetic house, associated with the root chakra and alchemical lead, suggests a major bottoming. In the grand scheme of the precession of the equinoxes and solstices, let's hope that 2020 was a low point preparing for a turnaround to cheerier times as Jupiter and Saturn transit through Aquarius in 2021. However, Saturn is not exactly the most cheer-inducing planet, and, to be honest, Aquarius has its share of problematic qualities as well, including what appears to be runaway technology.

When concerned with the ending of major cycles, like what we experienced at the end of the Capricorn extravaganza, it is important to evaluate how drastic the death must be prior to the rebirth. It is clear that many cycles are ending at this time, including a large one related to Pluto, at the end of the twelfth Hermetic sign, Capricorn. In terms of the ending of the Hindu Kali Yuga, one way of telling the story is that Kali needs to thoroughly destroy the old before the new can be reborn. Abrupt climate change could arguably range from simple disturbance to serious extinctions. I guess we will just need to see how Kali plays this one. Ha!

It is impressive that so many important conjunctions between Jupiter and the outer planets emphasize the first few accumulating signs of the Hermetic houses. For example, Neptune in his ruling sign, Pisces, gives the second chakra plenty of watery flowing and merging. Chiron and Eris in Aries, along with plenty of other transits through the third chakra fire sign, add lots of intense energy. Pluto's square to Eris makes the fire radioactively intense. Let's hope that Chiron can help the fires have some healing effects; fire can do that.

Giant Jupiter meeting up with radical Uranus in 2024 promises to be the beginning of an intense cycle of Promethean competition. Fortunately, Vacca/Taurus and the fourth heart chakra are the battlefield for this struggle. The heart center, represented by a green six-pointed star, is a balance point and can symbolize oneness, in which case the game is over. The remainder of Jupiter's transits through mercurial Gemini and participation in the alchemical union while transiting silvery Cancer and golden Leo suggests brilliant enlightenment, if humanity survives, that is! The year 2026 has a dangerous-looking stellium in fiery Aries to negotiate.

RARE PERIOD
OF ALL THE PLANETS
TRANSITING THEIR HOME SIGNS

Beginning November 5, 1983, when Pluto first transited into Scorpio, through March 30, 2025, when Neptune will complete transiting Pisces, those born in this period will have had all the planets completely transit their home signs:

Jupiter, Mars, and the faster inner planets all made several transits of their home signs.

Saturn transited Capricorn from 1988 to 1991 (2.5 years) and did so again from 2017 to 2020.

Uranus transited Aquarius from 1996 to 2003 (7 years).

Neptune, which began transiting Pisces in 2011, will complete transiting Pisces in 2025 (14 years).

Pluto transited Scorpio from 1983 to 1995 (12 years).

If Eris is eventually assigned as related to or co-ruler of Vacca/Taurus, as the Alchemical Tantric Arrangement of the zodiac suggests, then after entering Aries on January 10, 1927, and transiting that sign for 117 years, it will enter its home sign of Vacca/Taurus on June 4, 2044. If it happens to be assigned to Aries, then most of us have been able to experience her full ruling glory for all of our lives.

It is interesting to consider what this means for the folks who are living through this period and receiving the full symbolic force of all the planets completely transiting their home signs. I say again that clearly the alchemists of old knew, or intuited, the importance of astrological timing and symbolism in their "royal art," showing us how the celestial wisdom of astrology can point us toward a practical path to enlightenment.

Annotated Bibliography

Baker, Frederick, and Jeannine Parvati Baker. *Conscious Conception: Elemental Journey through the Labyrinth of Sexuality.* Berkeley, CA: Freestone and North Atlantic Books, 1986. A rich compilation about fertile sexuality, including myth, symbol, and the astrology of conception.

Brown, Norman Oliver. *Hermes the Thief.* Madison: University of Wisconsin Press, 1947. Scholarly and insightful hybrid of the classics and Freudian psychology.

Burckhardt, Titus. *Alchemy: Science of the Cosmos, Science of the Soul.* Translated by William Stoddart. Baltimore, MD: Penguin Books, 1974. This was my first introduction to alchemy, and it is a great one. It comes close to making the connection of the planets and the chakras.

Byrnes, Ronald Laurence. *Jesus and the Holy Shroud.* Bloomington, IN: First Books, 2002. An introductory presentation of occult historical astrology.

Castleden, Rodney. *The Knossos Labyrinth.* New York: Routledge, 1990. A thorough tour through the mythology, history, and archaeology of the great Labyrinth of Crete.

Clow, Barbara Hand. *Astrology and the Rising of Kundalini: The Transformative Power of Saturn, Chiron, and Uranus.* Rochester, VT: Bear & Company, 2013. Barbara is an excellent astrologer who also understands kundalini. Not surprisingly, she associates the same three planets that I do with the serpent power in her book.

Dass, Baba Hari. *Ashtanga Yoga Primer.* Santa Cruz, CA: Sri Rama, 1981. A great primer for all the practical parts of meditating in tune with the Alchemical Tantric Arrangement.

———. *Path Unfolds: The Autobiography of Baba Hari Dass.* Santa Cruz, CA: Sri Rama, 2019. An inspiring story of extreme austerity and living the actual life of a Himalayan yogi.

———. *The Yoga Sutras of Patanjali Samadhi Pada.* Santa Cruz, CA: Sri Rama, 1999. Translation and commentary by Baba Hari Dass.

De Lubicz, R. A. Schwaller. *The Egyptian Miracle.* Rochester, VT: Inner Traditions, 1985. Clarifies Egypt's spiritual primacy.

de Santillana, Giorgio, and Hertha von Dechend. *Hamlet's Mill: An Essay Investigating the Origins of Human Knowledge and Its Transmission through Myth.* Boston, MA: Nonpareil, 1977. This title says it well. A *wow!* book on myth, astronomy, and precession of the equinoxes.

Eisler, Riane. *The Chalice and the Blade.* San Francisco: Harper, 1988. Huge paradigm changer for recognizing gender blindness in history, archaeology, and daily life.

Firstenberg, Arthur. *The Invisible Rainbow: A History of Electricity and Life.* Santa Fe, NM: AGB Press, 2017. Valuable for understanding how electricity is affecting our health, especially in terms of modern technology and the body electric.

Frabricius, Johannes. *Alchemy: The Medieval Alchemists and Their Royal Art.* Copenhagen: Rosenkilde and Bagger, 1976. Written from the perspective of depth psychology.

Frawley, David. *Astrology of the Seers.* Twin Lakes, WI: Lotus Press, 2000. Vedic astrologer with an appreciation of the value of combining Eastern and Western astrology.

Grasse, Ray. *Eastern Systems for Western Astrologers.* Newburyport, MA: Red Wheel/Weiser, 1997. An anthology including Ray Grasse's thorough presentation of "Astrology and the Chakras."

Greene, Liz. *Saturn: A New Look at an Old Devil.* New York: Samuel Weiser, 1976. Groundbreaking psychology and astrology of this much misunderstood planet.

Grossinger, Richard. *Dark Pool of Light: Reality and Consciousness.* Vol. 2. *Consciousness in the Psychophysical and Psychic Ranges.* Berkeley, CA:

North Atlantic Books, 2012. More of Richard's brilliant and poetic exploration of consciousness. It includes an insightful psychic tour through
the chakras.

Harness, Dennis M. *The Nakshatras*. Twin Lakes, WI: Lotus Press, 1999.
Simple and easy to use.

Harrison, Jane Ellen. *Mythology*. New York: Harcourt/Harbinger Books,
1963. Refreshing gender-balanced scholarship.

————. *Prolegomena to the Study of Greek Religion and Mythology*. San
Bernadino, CA: Forgotten Books, 2012. A brilliant presentation of
fair gender-sensitive mythology. First printed in Cambridge, England,
in 1903.

Hickey, Isabel. *Astrology: A Cosmic Science*. Watertown, MA: Fellowship
House, 1970. One of my favorites for the basics, with a "cosmic" touch.

Hillman, James. *The Dream and the Underworld*. New York: Harper & Row,
1979.

————. *Pan and the Nightmare*. Dallas, TX: Spring, 1972.

————. *Revisioning Psychology*. New York: HarperCollins, 1975. Primary
source for archetypal psychology. Professor Hillman was highly influential in my psychology education, and this book was a major text in my
Masters program in archetypal psychology at Sonoma State University.

Homer. *The Homeric Hymns*. Translated by Charles Boer. Dallas, TX: Spring,
1979. Mythic prayers.

Jenkins, John Major. Jenkin's books are inspiring as were my discussions with
him on a 2010 pilgrimage through Guatemala and Izapa, Mexico.

————. *Galactic Alignment*. Rochester, VT: Bear & Company, 2002.

————. *The 2012 Story*. New York: Tarcher/Penguin, 2009.

Jones, Marc Edmund. *The Sabian Symbols*. Stanwood, WA: Sabian, 1966. The
original degree symbol system.

Jung, Carl G. *The Collected Works of Carl Jung*. Princeton, NJ: Princeton
University Press, 1953. See especially the volumes on alchemy, astrology,
mandalas, Hermes/Mercurius, and numerology.

————. *The Psychology of Kundalini Yoga*. Princeton, NJ: Princeton University
Press, 1996. Edited by Sonu Shamdasani, with an introduction and notes
from Jung's 1932 seminar.

Kerényi, Károly. Classic mythology from the perspective of a brilliant scholar
who writes in the style of a believer.

———. *Apollo: The Wind, the Spirit, and the God.* Dallas, TX: Spring, 1983

———. *Athene: Virgin and Mother in Greek Religion.* Dallas, TX: Spring, 1978.

———. *Goddesses of Sun and Moon.* Dallas, TX: Spring, 1979. Brilliance and darkness.

———. *The Gods of the Greeks.* London: Thames and Hudson, 1976. A classic of scholarship by a friend of the divinities. This book was recommended to our Master's class by James Hillman and has been my favorite book on mythology.

———. *Hermes Guide of Souls.* Zurich: Spring, 1976.

Lawlor, Robert. *The Geometry of the End of Time.* Melbourne: Wizarts, 2015. Brilliantly interweaves yugas and precession with mathematical precision.

Lopez-Pedraza, Rafael. *Hermes and His Children.* Dallas, TX: Spring, 1977. Archetypal psychotherapy of the wonderful and bizarre.

Martineau, John. *A Little Book of Coincidence: In the Solar System.* New York: Walker, 2001. Packed with beautiful patterns of the planets.

McKenna, Terence. *The Invisible Landscape.* New York: Seabury Press, 1975. Adventures in consciousness by this unique ethnobotanist and friend.

Narby, Jeremy. *The Cosmic Serpent.* New York: Jeremy Tarcher/Putnam, 1998. A story of awakening to the Cosmic Serpent and its sister in the DNA molecule. A key resource.

Norman, Garth. *Izapa Sacred Space.* American Fork, UT: ARCON, 2012. Garth was the primary archaeologist at the amazing proto-Mayan site of Izapa, presiding over a major winter solstice 2012 celebration event on site in southern Mexico.

Oswalt, Sabine. *Concise Encyclopedia of Greek and Roman Mythology.* Chicago: Follett Larousse, 1969. Handy small-sized and complete reference.

Parkyn, Chetan. *Human Design.* Novato, CA: New World Library, 2009. A basic guide to the system based on several traditions, among them astrology, I Ching, and acupuncture.

Prime, Ranchor. *Hinduism and Ecology Seeds of Truth.* Delhi: Motilal Banarsidass, 1996. Demonstrates strong elements of evolution and ecology in Hinduism and Indian myth.

Radin, Dean. *Supernormal: Science, Yoga, and the Evidence for Extraordinary Psychic Abilities.* New York: Deepak Chopra Books, 2013. This book has been helpful in making more sense of the siddhis and their Western equivalents.

Rudhyar, Dane. Many books by this genius are classics; I have read as many as I could find.

———. *An Astrological Mandala*. New York: Vintage Books, 1974.

———. *An Astrological Study of Psychological Complexes*. Berkeley, CA: Shambhala, 1976.

———. *Astrology and the Modern Psyche: An Astrologer Looks at Depth Psychology*. Petaluma, CA: Crcs, 1976.

———. *The Astrology of America's Destiny*. New York: Vintage Books, 1975.

———. *The Pulse of Life*. Berkeley, CA: Shambhala, 1970.

Schneider, Michael S. *A Layman's guide to Constructing the Universe*. New York: HarperCollins, 1995. Wonderful stories of numbers and their examples in nature.

Seltzer, Henry. *The Tenth Planet*. Bournemouth, UK: Wessex Astrologer, 2015. The foundational astrology of Eris. I also enjoy using his astrological software, "Time Passages," as utilized throughout this book.

Sitler, Robert. *The Living Maya*. Berkeley, CA: North Atlantic Books, 2010. An author and linguist, Sitler was our interpreter in Guatemala. This book has the perfect balance of scholarship and personal viewpoints.

Spretnak, Charlene. *Lost Goddesses of Early Greece*. Berkeley, CA: Moon Books, 1978. A lovely retelling of several Greek goddess myths from a matriarchal perspective.

Tarnas, Richard. *Cosmos and Psyche*. New York: Penguin, 2007. A scholarly work by a noted historian giving astrology an authoritative foundation.

———. *Prometheus the Awakener*. Thompson, CT: Spring Publications, 2018. This is the core and essence of his larger work listed above.

Trungpa, Chogyam. *Cutting through Spiritual Materialism*. Berkeley, CA: Shambhala, 1973. Essential Buddhism, from basics to advanced, in plain terms.

Walker, Barbara. *Woman's Encyclopedia of Myths and Secrets*. New York: HarperCollins, 1983. An amazing feminist education.

West, John Anthony. *Serpent in the Sky*. New York: Julian Press, 1986. Presents a view of ancient Egypt that lovingly and intelligently demonstrates a vast wisdom highly developed many millennia ago.

Wind, Edgar. *Pagan Mysteries in the Renaissance*. New York: W. W. Norton,

1968. The subtitle says it well: "An exploration of philosophical and mystical sources of iconography in Renaissance art." A wonderful classic.

Yan, Johnson F. *DNA and the I Ching: The Tao of Life*. Berkeley, CA: North Atlantic Books, 1991. Good introduction to mathematics and geometry with ancient background.

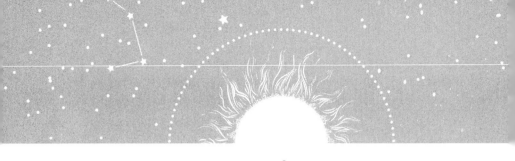

Index

Numbers in *italics* preceded by *pl.* refer to color plate numbers.

About the Author

My journey into astrology began initially through the writings of Carl Jung, whose work I read while in the humanistic psychology program at University of California, Santa Cruz. I discovered that a recognized authority actually appreciated astrology as a valid tool for psychology. At that time, I was also fortunate to meet and study with great teachers in Santa Cruz, including psychologists Gregory Bateson and Norman O. Brown, and spiritual teachers, including Zen master Suzuki Roshi and Himalayan yoga master Baba Hari Dass, with whom I continued studying yoga. Babaji gave me the name of Vishnu Dass and later called me Paran Purusha. In Santa Cruz, I also met iconic astrologer Lewis Fein, who was my first astrology teacher.

In the 1960s and '70s we had a warm and willing group of young local astrologers, including Marcia Stark, Jeannine Parvati, William Lonsdale, and Robert Cole, who shared astrological insights and traded reading one another's charts. Jeannine and I can be credited with introducing Rob Brezsny to James Hillman's books. I read all of Dane Rudhyar's books I could find and was able to attend a wonderfully inspiring workshop he presented in San Francisco, along with José Argüelles. The workshop was focused on his newly published book, *The Planetarization of Consciousness,* while José and his wife, Miriam, presented their artwork on mandalas and the subtle body. This workshop made a lasting impression on my life and studies.

I have maintained a professional astrology practice for more than

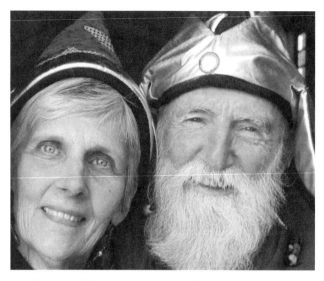

Claire and Rico in their astrologer hats in 2012

forty years and was the featured astrologer on the Linda Goodman website. I am presently interested in integrating Western astrological counseling with ayurveda, Vastu, jyotish, yoga, and other Vedic wisdom traditions. I studied intensively with Vaidyanatha Ganapati, one of India's premier *sthapatis* (temple architects) in the Vastu Shastra tradition, and his dedicated American student Ronald Quinn.

My wife, Claire, and I have been studying ayurveda with Vaidya Yashashree since 2008. Together we traveled to Guatemala in 2010, where we studied the Mayan calendar with Mayan elders and scholars. Later that year, we traveled to India to learn more about the ayurvedic treatment of serious diseases. Claire has introduced me to many wonderful folks in the field of radical nonduality, including Tony Parsons, Naho Owada, Andreas Mueller, Jim Newman, and Prasanna, as well as the occult astrologer Ronald L. Byrnes.